THE 30-MINUTE
FIBROMYALGIA COOKBOOK

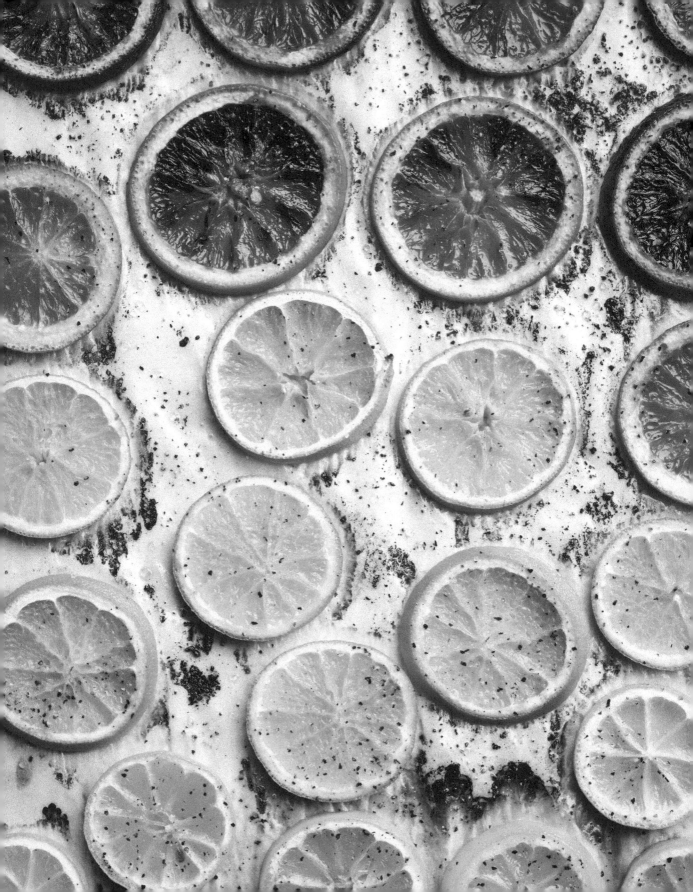

THE 30-MINUTE

FIBROMYALGIA

COOKBOOK

75 Quick and Easy Anti-Inflammatory Recipes

BONNIE NASAR, RDN

Photography by Iain Bagwell

ROCKRIDGE PRESS

Interior and Cover Designer: Monica Cheng
Art Producer: Meg Baggott
Editor: Nadina Persaud
Production Editor: Nora Milman

Photography © 2020 Iain Bagwell.
Food styling by Katelyn Hardwick.

Author photo courtesy of Juliet Nasar.

ISBN: Print 978-1-64739-686-2
eBook 978-1-64739-421-9

R0

In blessed memory of my dear father,
the esteemed rheumatologist Dr. Mori Schwartzberg.
I felt your presence with every recipe created
and every word written.

Avocado-Mint Sorbet ▸ page 99

CONTENTS

INTRODUCTION

Nutrition is a tricky business with a lot of information circulating that is not always based on sound science. For registered dietitians, a large part of our job is weeding through the nutrition myths and separating fact from fiction for our patients. Sometimes clinical studies are scarce and we have to think outside the box, relying on what limited research we can find and the anecdotal evidence from our private practices. I am forever grateful to have learned my critical thinking skills from my father, Dr. Mori Schwartzberg (may his memory be a blessing). As a rheumatologist, he treated many patients with fibromyalgia at a time when most doctors believed it was a psychiatric condition. He was advocating for his patients before advocating was even a trend. My father also instilled in me, from a very young age, a love for nutrition and an understanding of how the foods we eat affect our health.

I remember hearing my father talk about fibromyalgia when I was very little. He would have stacks of research articles all around him, reading intently, confounded by this unusual constellation of symptoms that he was seeing in his practice. Fibromyalgia, like most chronic pain conditions, remains difficult to understand and therefore difficult to treat. But there is hope! Most experts believe in a multidisciplinary approach, focusing on symptom management. In this book we will focus on how one aspect of this approach, nutrition, can help decrease symptoms and increase quality of life.

My work with chronic pain patients started with my own chronic pain issues. When I realized that my symptoms were affecting my ability to function in daily life, I put my expertise and training as a registered dietitian to work. I read all the evidenced-based research articles I could get my hands on. I learned about pain-signaling pathways and how they can be affected by the foods we eat and the chemicals and hormones we release to digest them. My research led me to develop a way of eating that decreased my chronic pain, brain fog, and fatigue—and left me with a mission. I wanted to help others who, like me, had to put their lives on hold due to chronic pain.

With renewed energy, I left my job as a consultant dietitian and opened a virtual private practice for chronic pain patients. I developed a method to start slowly, reducing the foods that aggravated symptoms in my pain warriors while adding nutrient-dense beneficial ones. My patients responded beautifully to this nutrition protocol. The recipes in this book are created based on my experiences with my patients.

A lot of fibromyalgia warriors want to use dietary interventions to feel better but worry about their ability to cook for extended periods of time, using up precious energy. The recipes in this book are carefully curated to focus on cooking nutritious, pain-relieving meals in under 30 minutes, with lots of shortcuts that can save you time while maximizing taste. Many meals can be made in advance and even frozen for those days you feel like you need to take it easy. Lots of tips and tidbits are also included to make your kitchen more fibro-friendly. I hope the information gathered here will help make your days more manageable. I couldn't be more excited about taking this journey with you!

Lemon-Oregano Chicken ▸ *page 90*

Chapter 1

🌿

FINDING FIBROMYALGIA RELIEF WITH FOOD

There are plenty of cookbooks for meals in a hurry, and even a few for fibromyalgia warriors. However, a book with mouthwatering recipes in under 30 minutes specifically for the fibromyalgia community did not exist . . . until now! This book is a handy guide for using your time in the kitchen wisely. It combines the latest research with delicious, nutrient-dense ingredients and simple directions for healthy, easy meals. Let's start by covering some basics.

About Fibromyalgia

While chronic pain conditions were first officially recognized in 1904, the term "fibromyalgia" was not used until 1976. The American College of Rheumatology published diagnostic criteria to help physicians identify fibromyalgia in 1990. Even now, the medical community does not always take this syndrome seriously. According to a 2010 patient survey from *BMC Health Services Research*, it takes an average of 2.3 years and 3.7 doctors for patients to get properly diagnosed.

Part of the problem is that there is no test to definitively diagnose fibromyalgia. Patients must seek out physicians familiar with the syndrome in order to get a proper diagnosis.

Fibromyalgia is painful; those with it suffer from tender spots over muscles, joints, and skin that feel painful when touched. They often have debilitating fatigue, potentially due to poor sleep quality, and difficulty thinking clearly. Other medical issues often arise with fibromyalgia, including depression, bowel and bladder irritability, migraines, and acid reflux.

What Causes Fibromyalgia?

As of the publishing of this book, the origin of fibromyalgia remains a mystery. This syndrome is relatively new and data is limited. What the researchers do know, however, is that certain factors can contribute to it. They include:

GENETICS

Fibromyalgia appears to run in some families. Those with a first-degree relative (defined as a parent, full sibling, or child) who has been diagnosed with fibromyalgia are eight times more likely to be diagnosed with it as well.

STRESS

Symptoms tend to present during or after traumatic events. This can include daily stressors as well as acute events, whether physical or emotional.

AUTOIMMUNE DISEASES

While fibromyalgia is not currently considered an autoimmune disorder, those diagnosed with autoimmune diseases have an increased risk of fibromyalgia. These can include lupus, rheumatoid arthritis, and others.

While the exact pathway of fibromyalgia in the body has eluded us, the best explanation of what fibromyalgia feels like for a person suffering from the condition is that the neurons in the body that feel pain somehow get turned on "high" and the sensation of pain is amplified. One way to manage these symptoms is through diet.

Soothing Symptoms with Food

A multidisciplinary approach is the most effective way to treat fibromyalgia. Physical therapy, medication, stress management, sleep hygiene, and nutrition therapy are integral parts of this team effort. Recent research suggests that focusing on nutrition can reduce the symptoms of fibromyalgia. Some foods are thought to be inherently inflammatory and excitatory to the body, contributing to pain, fatigue, and brain fog. Supporting your body with the right kinds of nutrients and avoiding certain foods can increase your quality of life.

This book will introduce you to a whole-foods approach to nutrition, focusing on replacing inflammatory foods with nutrient-dense ones. This supports your body's ability to calm, heal, and repair itself. Remember that team approach? Your organs are a team, too, and your gastrointestinal tract is the MVP. Nourish it!

This book is designed to provide information for fibromyalgia sufferers and is not a substitute for medical care. Please consult with your physician or registered dietitian if you have any concerns. If you have any food allergies or intolerances, make substitutions as needed.

Tools to Speed Things Up

- **Electric citrus juicer:** squeeze your lemons, limes, oranges, and other citruses quickly and easily

- **Immersion blender:** great for whipping up homemade dressings, smoothies, and creamy soups—all with less cleanup than a traditional blender

- **Jar opener:** the perfect gadget during flare-ups

- **Food processor:** chop food quickly using this appliance

- **Vegetable spiralizer:** an easy, sneaky way to replace some regular noodles with nutrient-rich vegetables

Foods for Healing

While peer-reviewed nutrition research is hard to find in fibromyalgia literature, a study published in 2000 in the *Scandinavian Journal of Rheumatology* suggests that a vegan way of eating might increase quality of life. It is not necessary to go completely vegan, but this study illustrates that eating a variety of fruits and vegetables daily can help you feel better. In my practice, I have found that many patients benefit from replacing sugary foods with more nutrient-dense plant-based foods. The recipes in this book are rich in fruits and vegetables, which means you are getting more bang for your buck when it comes to vitamins and minerals.

Here is a list of some important foods to include into your meals:

Almonds	Flaxseed	Salmon
Arugula	Hazelnuts	Sardines
Blueberries	Hemp seeds	Spinach
Broccoli	Kale	Strawberries
Brussels sprouts	Pumpkin seeds	Sunflower seeds
Carrots	Red cherries	Sweet potatoes

Foods to Avoid

Some studies show that fibromyalgia patients who improved their way of eating experienced a reduction of symptoms. Interestingly, these symptoms returned when their eating habits slid back into a standard American diet (SAD). SAD foods include highly processed and preserved items, sugary snacks, and nightshade vegetables. This seems to trigger symptoms. Try to avoid:

- Aged cheeses, such as cheddar and Parmesan; dairy in general has a more individualized effect, so it's best to discuss this with a physician or dietitian

- Artificial colors, flavors, and preservatives (check ingredients list)

- Aspartame (check ingredients list)

▻ FODMAPs (a group of sugars found in some foods: Fermentable Oligo-, Di-, Mono-saccharides And Polyols), if there is a known sensitivity

▻ Monosodium glutamate (MSG) (check ingredients list)

▻ Nightshade vegetables

Bell peppers   *Tomatoes*

Cayenne pepper   *White potatoes*

Eggplant

▻ Processed foods, which are anything boxed or bagged with long lists of ingredients, including preservatives and other difficult-to-pronounce items

Five Shortcuts to a Fine Meal

🖋 Buy precut veggies, either fresh or frozen. Frozen vegetables are preferable to canned, which typically have a higher sodium content and preservatives. Leafy greens, like kale and spinach, can also be purchased precut, pre-washed, and bagged.

🖋 Buy precooked items, always checking the ingredient list for foods to avoid. If the food comes with a sauce or dressing, throw it out and make your own at home.

🖋 Chop using a food processor. It won't be as pretty as if you sliced by hand, but it will still taste the same!

🖋 For foods that you do want to look nice, you can use a mandoline slicer. Take care to use a hand guard and be extra careful when cleaning the slicer.

🖋 Consider prepping and freezing onions, garlic cloves, and spices in batches. Wash, chop, and freeze individual portions in a silicone chocolate mold or ice cube tray. Store the frozen portions in an airtight freezer bag or container.

Kitchen and Pantry Staples

A well-stocked kitchen makes cooking that much easier. The goal is getting nutritious food on the table fast, and having the right ingredients on hand is required to do so.

Fridge

▶ **Avocados:** A great source of good fat that you can dice and add to salads or other meals, make guacamole, or throw in a smoothie.

▶ **Broccoli slaw or shredded cabbage/Brussels sprouts:** Great for a salad shortcut!

▶ **Collard greens:** A little-known secret about collards is that they can be used instead of bread for those who are sensitive to wheat or gluten. Dip these leaves in boiling water, then in ice water to make a great gluten-free sandwich wrap.

▶ **Hummus:** Pureed chickpeas that you can use as a dip, sauce, or spread. Pick up a container at the grocery store if you'd rather not make your own.

▶ **Fresh herbs (parsley, dill, rosemary, cilantro):** Complex sauces take time, but fresh herbs just need a wash and a chop to elevate the flavor of any simple dish. Sprinkle them on top of just about anything you make.

▶ **Lemons and limes:** These flavorful, vitamin C–rich powerhouses are also a natural preservative! I recommend an inexpensive electric citrus juicer for those who may find it too painful to squeeze them.

▶ **Zucchini noodles:** Buy them spiralized if you don't have a spiralizer or mandoline slicer.

Freezer

▶ **Beyond Beef:** The best-tasting vegan replacement for ground meat. While this is technically processed, it is still a better alternative for those looking to eat less red meat. The preservatives used by the company are all-natural.

▶ **Frozen herbs:** If you happen to find frozen herbs, buy them! They are usually sold in prechopped teaspoon-size servings.

- **Frozen vegetables and fruits:** Frozen produce is actually quite healthy; the flash-freezing upon harvesting helps retain all the nutrients, making them a safe alternative to canned vegetables that are loaded with preservatives, or fresh produce that spoils quickly.

- **Precooked brown rice and quinoa:** A huge help on a busy day.

Pantry

- **Avocado oil:** Avocado oil is best for higher-temperature cooking, like frying, because of its higher smoking point.

- **Canned beans:** Ideally these should be organic and BPA-free.

- **Extra-virgin olive oil:** EVOO is great for drizzling and sautéing. This should be your go-to for lower-temperature cooking, such as sautéing, because it has a low smoking point.

- **Flaxseed:** High in omega-3 fatty acids, these add a nutty flavor. Ground flaxseed can also be used as an egg substitute.

- **Hemp seeds:** A great vegan protein, hemp seeds are earthy and nutty in flavor.

- **Nutritional yeast.** This is an excellent addition to any savory dish for depth of flavor without dairy.

- **Oats:** Not only are oats packed with fiber, but a warm bowl is soothing for the body and soul.

- **Onions and garlic:** These are a staple for flavor in many dishes. They also keep for one to three months depending on storage methods, so stock up!

- **Organic vegetable broth:** You can make your own or pick some up from the store.

- **Quinoa:** The edible seed of this whole grain can be sweet or savory, and it cooks faster than rice.

In a Pinch

▲

The recipes included in this book are fast and easy. For those days when making a meal *still* seems impossible, use this simple system.

Choose items from this list of ingredients:

- A protein (the size of a deck of playing cards)

- Vegetables (as much as you want)

- An oil (1 to 2 tablespoons)

- Spices and/or dried herbs (a few shakes)

Sauté the veggies and protein in oil until fully cooked, then sprinkle with your spices and herbs. Cook for another minute or two, and you're done!

Some go-to snack ideas:

- Sliced apple with nut butter

- Carrot sticks with hummus

- Organic vegetable broth

- Sliced cucumbers with a schmear of plant-based cream cheese topped with lox

- Celery sticks with guacamole

Eight Tips for Relief

1. **Sleep hygiene.** Eliminate screen time about two hours before bedtime. Aim for at least eight hours of sleep per night. Begin a bedtime routine and do it each night.

2. **Exercise.** Physical exercise is good for your body and mind and can help reduce symptoms.

3. **Eat a diet rich in fruits and vegetables.** This book has you covered!

4. **Nutrition supplements.** Ask your doctor or registered dietitian for specific recommendations.

5. **Stress management.** Try meditation, yoga, flotation pods, and Himalayan breathing rooms. You can even do an app-based relaxation program from your smartphone. A hobby can be a great stress reliever, too. It's important to know when to slow down and take it easy!

6. **Heat packs or ice packs.** Utilize either of these depending on which works better for you. Studies indicate that both can be helpful.

7. **Medical massages.** These can help eliminate muscle soreness and stress. Find someone who is knowledgeable about fibromyalgia. Check with your insurance provider to see if they offer coverage.

8. **Medication options.** Don't be afraid to discuss medication with your physician. There are nonopioid options that can offer some relief.

The 30-Minute Recipes

The recipes in this book use a variety of nutrient-packed fruits and vegetables that are good for the body in every way. Lean proteins and unsaturated fats are emphasized. All the included recipes can be made in 30 minutes or less with a few small (but worthy) exceptions, regardless of your cooking skills. You'll spend less time in the kitchen and more time enjoying your healthier lifestyle!

This book focuses on a Mediterranean style of eating—heavy on the vegetables, berries, good fats and fishes, and lean proteins. The goal is to minimize processed food items and artificial ingredients, while embracing whole foods and whole grains. Sometimes, for the sake of convenience, frozen or canned items will be specified.

My objective is to show you how to properly nourish your body quickly and with minimal effort. Each recipe includes a tip with ideas on substitutions or storing foods properly. Recipes will have the following labels: Five Ingredients or Less (not including common ingredients such as salt, pepper, water, or oil), Freezer-Friendly, Make-Ahead, One-Pot, and Vegetarian or Vegan.

Chai-Spiced Quinoa Breakfast Bowl ▸ **page 26**

Chapter 2

🌿

BEVERAGES AND BREAKFAST

FOUR-SEED NO-OATMEAL

**MAKE-AHEAD,
ONE-POT, VEGAN**

Serves 1
Prep time: 3 minutes
Cook time: 2 minutes

½ cup water

2 tablespoons almond flour

2 tablespoons white
    sesame seeds

2 tablespoons unsalted
    sunflower seeds, shelled

2 tablespoons chia seeds

2 tablespoons flaxseed meal

½ teaspoon ground cinnamon

½ teaspoon maple syrup

Pinch salt

½ teaspoon vanilla extract

Hearty and fragrant with a warm note of cinnamon spice, this four-seed no-oatmeal is a treat any time of the day but is particularly suitable for busy mornings. Sesame, sunflower, chia seeds, and flaxseed combine to create a porridge packed with an array of vitamins and minerals along with inflammation-reducing omega-3 fatty acids, plant-based protein, and fiber to keep you feeling full until lunch.

1. In a microwave-safe bowl, combine the water, almond flour, sesame seeds, sunflower seeds, chia seeds, flaxseed, cinnamon, maple syrup, and salt. Stir to mix.

2. Microwave on high for 2 minutes. Stir to eliminate any hot spots and add the vanilla. Let cool for 1 minute. Serve warm.

Tip: Swap the water with your favorite milk (dairy or plant-based) for a creamier porridge. For a smoother texture, substitute almond flour for the sunflower seeds.

....

Per serving: Calories: 510; Total fat: 40g; Total carbs: 26g; Fiber: 20g; Sugar: 3g; Protein: 18g; Sodium: 167mg

ALMOND MUG CAKE WITH BLUEBERRY CHIA JAM

ONE-POT, VEGAN

Serves 1
Prep time: 3 minutes
Cook time: 4 minutes

⅓ cup almond flour

⅓ teaspoon baking powder

2 teaspoons ground flaxseed

1 teaspoon maple syrup

1¾ tablespoons unsweetened
   vanilla almond milk

1¾ tablespoons water

1 teaspoon coconut oil,
   softened

⅛ teaspoon cinnamon

Pinch salt

Blueberry-Lemon Chia Jam
   (page 113)

Mug cakes are an easy and delicious way to feel like you are eating dessert for breakfast. This one is no exception! Decadent blueberry jam adds the perfect fruit accompaniment.

1. In a microwave-safe bowl, combine the almond flour, baking powder, flaxseed, maple syrup, almond milk, water, oil, cinnamon, and salt.

2. Microwave on high for 1½ minutes. Carefully remove the mug from the microwave (the handle will be hot). Put a dollop of the jam on top. Let cool for 1 minute.

Tip: To melt the coconut oil, microwave it in the mug before adding the other ingredients. For a no-sugar version, use Lakanto maple-flavored syrup.

Per serving: Calories: 299; Total fat: 25g; Total carbs: 14g; Fiber: 6g; Sugar: 6g; Protein: 9g; Sodium: 341mg

BAKED OATMEAL WITH BERRIES

FREEZER-FRIENDLY, MAKE-AHEAD, VEGAN

Serves 6

Prep time: 5 minutes

Cook time: 20 minutes

Olive oil cooking spray

2 cups rolled oats

2 cups unsweetened almond milk

2 tablespoons maple syrup

½ cup unsweetened applesauce

1 teaspoon cinnamon

2 tablespoons chia seeds

2 cups frozen mixed berries

Pinch salt

¼ cup sliced almonds

This breakfast is a hearty oatmeal that you can make ahead and reheat the next morning so there is no prep work when you wake up! This recipe is packed with fiber and antioxidants. Chia seeds are an excellent source of omega-3 fatty acids, which are known to decrease inflammation.

1. Preheat the oven to 400°F. Spray an 8-inch square baking pan with cooking spray.

2. In a bowl, combine the oats, almond milk, maple syrup, applesauce, cinnamon, chia seeds, berries, and salt. Stir until thoroughly mixed.

3. Pour the mixture into the greased baking pan. Bake for 20 minutes or until all the liquid is absorbed.

4. Divide into bowls and sprinkle with sliced almonds.

Tip: Make this dish in the beginning of the week and reheat in the mornings. It will keep well in a covered dish for 3 to 5 days in the refrigerator. This dish can also be frozen in individual portions. You can replace the almonds with any nut or seed of your choice.

Per serving: Calories: 214; Total fat: 6g; Total carbs: 34g; Fiber: 7g; Sugar: 10g; Protein: 6g; Sodium: 91mg

GOLDEN TURMERIC LATTE

MAKE-AHEAD, ONE-POT, VEGETARIAN

Serves 2
Prep time: 3 minutes
Cook time: 5 minutes

1 tablespoon grated fresh ginger, peeled, or 1 teaspoon ginger powder

1 cup unsweetened vanilla coconut milk

¾ cup water

1 teaspoon powdered turmeric

1 tablespoon honey

½ teaspoon cinnamon

2 teaspoons coconut oil

A drink with this golden color is like having a cup of sunshine to begin your day! Some studies indicate that turmeric, full of anti-inflammatory properties, is as powerful as ibuprofen. In a 2014 study published in Clinical Interventions in Aging, *patients with knee osteoarthritis were split into two groups. One group was given curcuma, the active ingredient in turmeric, and the other group was given ibuprofen. Both groups had significant similar reductions in pain and stiffness, but the curcuma group had fewer gastrointestinal side effects. While more research is needed, these results are very promising.*

1. If using fresh ginger, wrap the ginger in cheesecloth and squeeze it over a small pot. Discard the grated ginger after squeezing. If using powdered ginger, skip to step 2.

2. In a small pot, combine the ginger, coconut milk, water, turmeric, honey, cinnamon, and oil. Heat over medium-high heat until boiling, then lower to a simmer, stirring constantly. Cook for 3 to 5 minutes.

continued...

GOLDEN TURMERIC LATTE *continued*

3. Turn off the heat. Use an immersion blender or milk frother to get some air into the liquid, taking care not to let it splash out.

4. Pour into a mug and serve.

Tip: For an extra boost, add a scoop of protein powder. To make this vegan and/or sugar-free, use monk fruit sweetener instead of honey. Turmeric can stain, so be sure to clean everything carefully afterward.

Per serving: Calories: 104; Total fat: 7g; Total carbs: 11g; Fiber: 1g; Sugar: 9g; Protein: <1g; Sodium: 14mg

CINNAMON-AVOCADO SMOOTHIE

FIVE INGREDIENTS OR LESS, ONE-POT, VEGAN

*Serves **4***
*Prep time: **5 minutes***
*Cook time: **1 minute***

4 cups unsweetened almond milk

1 avocado

2 teaspoons vanilla extract

4 tablespoons maple syrup

Juice of 1 lemon or 2 tablespoons bottled lemon juice

½ cup ice cubes

This smoothie gets its richness from an unusual source—an avocado—rather than the more typical banana. Potassium is an important nutrient for helping muscles and nerves function properly, and avocados actually have more potassium per serving than bananas. Low levels of potassium can lead to fatigue and weakness. Avocados also have an abundance of insoluble fiber, which is great for keeping the digestive tract moving and preventing constipation. This smoothie tastes great and offers a satisfying creaminess that will keep you full all morning.

1. Place the almond milk, avocado, vanilla, maple syrup, lemon juice, and ice in a blender.

2. Blend on high for 30 to 60 seconds until completely smooth.

3. Pour into glasses and serve.

Tip: For a smoothie bowl, use 3 cups of almond milk to get a pudding-like consistency before adding toppings such as granola and fresh fruit. For a no-sugar option, substitute Lakanto maple-flavored syrup for regular maple syrup.

Per serving: Calories: 153; Total fat: 8g; Total carbs: 19g; Fiber: 2g; Sugar: 13g; Protein: 2g; Sodium: 176mg

FROZEN CHERRY SMOOTHIE

**FIVE INGREDIENTS OR
LESS, ONE-POT, VEGAN**

Serves 1

Prep time: 2 minutes

Cook time: 1 minute

1 cup unsweetened vanilla
  almond milk

1 cup dark sweet frozen
  cherries

1 tablespoon chia seeds

Juice of ½ lime or
  1 tablespoon bottled
  lime juice

Cherries are a great source of vitamin C and have anti-inflammatory properties. According to a 2018 study published in Nutrients, *regular ingestion of cherry juice reduced blood pressure and pain, while improving sleep quality. Fibromyalgia often causes pain, which can make sleeping at night difficult, and poor sleep can increase pain levels, creating a vicious cycle of pain and exhaustion. This smoothie is great for the days where you wake up feeling "blah."*

1. Put the almond milk, cherries, chia seeds, and lime juice into a blender.

2. Blend on high for 30 to 60 seconds until completely smooth.

3. Pour into glasses and serve.

Tip: For a smoothie bowl, use ½ cup of almond milk to get a pudding-like consistency and add toppings such as granola and fresh fruit of your choice.

....

Per serving: Calories: 188; Total fat: 8g; Total carbs: 32g; Fiber: 8g; Sugar: 20g; Protein: 4g; Sodium: 172mg

FLOURLESS PUMPKIN MUFFINS

**FREEZER-FRIENDLY,
MAKE-AHEAD,
VEGETARIAN**

*Makes **12 muffins***
*Prep time: **5 minutes***
*Cook time: **22 minutes***

Coconut oil or avocado oil, for
  coating (optional)
¾ cup canned 100-percent
  pure pumpkin puree
1 cup creamy almond butter,
  no salt or sugar added
2 large eggs
1 heaping tablespoon
  maple syrup
2 teaspoons vanilla extract
1 teaspoon ground cinnamon
½ teaspoon baking soda
½ teaspoon ground ginger
¼ teaspoon ground nutmeg
⅛ teaspoon salt
¼ cup quick or
  old-fashioned oats

Packed with pumpkin flavor and topped with toasty oats, these flourless muffins are incredible. You are greeted by the aroma of baked pumpkin, and with the first bite will indulge in the sweet and spicy flavors. This recipe uses cinnamon and nutmeg for complexity, and ginger for an unexpected kick.

1. Preheat the oven to 350°F. Line a 12-cup muffin pan with paper liners or lightly coat it with coconut oil.

2. In a large bowl, combine the pumpkin, almond butter, eggs, maple syrup, vanilla, cinnamon, baking soda, ginger, nutmeg, and salt. Mix until smooth.

3. Evenly distribute the batter into the prepared muffin pan.

4. Sprinkle the top of each muffin with one teaspoon of oats.

5. Bake for 22 minutes or until golden brown and a toothpick comes out with moist crumbs when inserted in the center.

6. Let cool for 10 minutes before serving.

Tip: Swap almond butter with sunflower butter for nut-free pumpkin muffins. The muffins can be eaten immediately or stored in an airtight container or plastic bag and refrigerated for 1 week, or frozen for 3 months.

....

Per serving (1 muffin): Calories: 161; Total fat: 13g; Total carbs: 8g; Fiber: 3g; Sugar: 3g; Protein: 6g; Sodium: 90mg

—

MEDITERRANEAN SCRAMBLED EGGS

FIVE INGREDIENTS OR LESS, ONE-POT, VEGETARIAN

Serves 2
Prep time: 3 minutes
Cook time: 4 minutes

2 tablespoons extra-virgin olive oil

2 cups fresh baby spinach

4 eggs, beaten

12 Kalamata olives, pitted and sliced

Salt

Freshly ground black pepper

This breakfast packs in lots of vitamin-rich spinach, so you're getting a serving of veggies before you even start your day! The antioxidants in spinach help lower inflammation throughout the body when eaten on a regular basis. While the reputation of eggs seems to rise and fall regularly, the current evidence points to eggs as a good source of protein that can be part of a balanced diet. The general recommendation is to have no more than 1 or 2 eggs per day. These eggs combine the earthy flavor of spinach with the salty brine of olives to keep your taste buds happy. They can be served with gluten-free toast.

1. In a skillet, heat the oil over medium heat.

2. Add the spinach and cook for 1 to 2 minutes until wilted, stirring when needed. Add the eggs and olives and continue to mix until the eggs are cooked, about 2 minutes. Season with salt and pepper.

3. Divide between two plates.

Tip: Feel free to play around with different veggies like frozen chopped broccoli or peas. Shredded vegan cheese can also be added for more flavor. For a vegan option, instead of 4 eggs, use 1 cup of Just Egg (found in health food stores).

....

Per serving: Calories: 343; Total fat: 30g; Total carbs: 6g; Fiber: 1g; Sugar: 1g; Protein: 12g; Sodium: 593mg

AVOCADO-HUMMUS TOAST

FIVE INGREDIENTS OR LESS, ONE-POT, VEGAN

Serves 4

Prep time: 5 minutes

2 cups hummus

8 slices gluten-free bread, toasted

2 avocados, sliced or mashed

Juice of 1 lemon or 2 tablespoons bottled lemon juice

2 teaspoons everything bagel spice mix

Avocados are full of healthy fat that will keep you satiated. This recipe is super-simple to put together as long as you have the ingredients on hand. It's also a great breakfast option on days you just don't have the energy to cook. The lemon adds a tartness to the creamy avocado slices and blends perfectly with the hummus flavor, while the everything spice sprinkled on top adds depth of flavor and crunch.

1. Spread the hummus over the toast and top it with avocado.

2. Sprinkle the lemon juice and everything spice on top and serve immediately.

Tip: Have fun with different flavors of hummus—there are tons of flavors to choose from!

· · · · · · · · · · · · · · · · ·

Per serving: Calories: 573; Total fat: 31g; Total carbs: 55g; Fiber: 16g; Sugar: 7g; Protein: 12g; Sodium: 894mg

KALE AND QUINOA EGG MUFFINS

FIVE INGREDIENTS OR LESS, FREEZER-FRIENDLY, MAKE-AHEAD, VEGETARIAN

Makes 6 muffins

Prep time: 2 minutes, plus 15 if cooking the quinoa

Cook time: 15 to 17 minutes

1½ teaspoons avocado oil

1 cup cooked quinoa

3 cups chopped fresh kale leaves

¼ cup plus 1 tablespoon water, divided

7 eggs

1 tablespoon extra-virgin olive oil

½ teaspoon salt

Egg cups are a great make-ahead-and-reheat breakfast item. The added quinoa makes these eggs fluffy and delicious. You can also easily make this vegan by using an egg substitute. Eggs are an excellent source of protein for building and repairing muscles, and quinoa is rich in B vitamins, which are essential for energy production. Kale is a great source of calcium, especially for those that avoid dairy.

1. Preheat an oven to 350°F. Grease 6 cups of a muffin pan with avocado oil.

2. If you do not have precooked quinoa, cook the quinoa according to the package directions and measure out 1 cup.

3. Put the kale in a microwave-safe bowl and add 1 tablespoon of water. Cover and microwave for 2 minutes on high, until the kale is wilted.

4. Add the cooked quinoa to the kale and stir to combine. Scoop the mixture evenly into the prepared muffin cups.

5. Crack the eggs into a mixing bowl and whisk until the yolks and whites are combined. Add the remaining ¼ cup of water, the olive oil, and salt and mix again. Pour the egg mixture into the muffin cups over the quinoa-kale mixture.

6. Bake for 15 to 17 minutes, until the egg is cooked through. Remove from the oven and let cool slightly before serving.

Tip: Quinoa can be purchased cooked and frozen from some stores. You can also save leftovers for this purpose. These muffins can be made ahead of time and refrigerated in an airtight container for up to 3 days. They can also be frozen. For a vegan option, use ¼ cup of an egg substitute (found in health food stores) per 1 egg.

....

Per serving (1 muffin): Calories: 150; Total fat: 10g; Total carbs: 8g; Fiber: 1g; Sugar: 1g; Protein: 8g; Sodium: 208mg

CHAI-SPICED QUINOA BREAKFAST BOWL

VEGETARIAN

Serves 4
Prep time: 5 minutes
Cook time: 18 minutes

1 cup uncooked quinoa

2 cups water

3 chai tea bags,
   strings removed

2 cups unsweetened
   almond milk

1 tablespoon maple syrup
   or honey

1 cup halved frozen sweet
   cherries

1 fresh peach, pitted and diced

¼ cup dry toasted slivered
   almonds, unsalted

¼ cup unsweetened
   coconut yogurt

Chai-infused quinoa, cherries, peaches, and almonds are the stars of this incredibly energizing breakfast bowl. Cooking the quinoa in chai tea allows each kernel to be infused with its pungent flavor. Combining this quinoa with the fruit results in an aromatic morning meal. The peaches add beta-carotene, which is good for night vision, and vitamin C, essential for skin and connective tissue regeneration. Cherries contain melatonin, which can help with sleep regulation.

1. Rinse the quinoa, then drain.

2. Transfer the quinoa to a medium saucepan. Add the water and tea bags.

3. Bring to a boil, then simmer, covered, for 15 minutes or until all the liquid has absorbed.

4. Remove the tea bags and discard them. Fluff the quinoa with a fork.

5. Add the almond milk, maple syrup, cherries, and peach. Stir to combine.

6. Cook over medium heat for 3 minutes.

7. Remove from the heat and fold in the almonds.

8. Ladle into bowls and top each serving with
    1 tablespoon of yogurt.

Tip: If peaches are not in season, substitute with an additional
½ cup of cherries or any fresh or frozen fruit of choice. Quinoa is
perfectly cooked when the kernels appear to have popped open
and the germ is exposed. The germ looks like a fine strand.

Per serving: Calories: 270; Total fat: 8g; Total carbs: 43g;
Fiber: 5g; Sugar: 14g; Protein: 9g; Sodium: 91mg

Swiss Chard with Chickpeas and Allspice ▸ **page 38**

Chapter 3

✤

SIDES AND SALADS

CHOPPED MEDITERRANEAN SALAD WITH TAHINA DRESSING

VEGAN

Serves 4

Prep time: 10 minutes

FOR THE SALAD

4 cups chopped
romaine lettuce

1 cucumber

1 (15-ounce) can chickpeas,
drained and rinsed

⅓ cup pitted Kalamata olives,
coarsely chopped

½ red onion, finely chopped

2 tablespoons fresh
flat-leaf parsley

FOR THE DRESSING

¼ cup tahini

¼ cup water

Juice of 1 lemon or
2 tablespoons bottled
lemon juice

¼ teaspoon garlic powder

Kosher salt

Freshly ground black pepper

Easy to prepare and even easier to eat, this hearty and healthy Mediterranean salad has it all, including the inflammation super-duo that is chickpeas and Kalamata olives. A 2011 study published in the European Journal of Nutrition *indicated that a lower-calorie diet rich in legumes such as chickpeas helped reduce pro-inflammatory markers. The brined olives in this recipe contain oleocanthal, a compound believed to have an anti-inflammatory role similar to ibuprofen.*

TO MAKE THE SALAD

1. In a large bowl, combine the lettuce, cucumber, chickpeas, olives, red onion, and parsley.

TO MAKE THE DRESSING

2. In a small bowl, whisk together the tahini, water, lemon juice, garlic powder, and salt and pepper.

3. Pour the dressing over the salad and toss.

Tip: Use a small vegetable chopper for the cucumber, olives, and onions to cut prep time. Try using other leafy greens to mix things up. You can also swap the parsley for fresh mint to add a cool, refreshing note to the salad, or omit it entirely.

Per serving: Calories: 231; Total fat: 12g; Total carbs: 26g; Fiber: 8g; Sugar: 6g; Protein: 9g; Sodium: 371mg

ASPARAGUS WITH CREAMY AVOCADO SAUCE

FIVE INGREDIENTS OR LESS, VEGAN

Serves 4
Prep time: 1 minute
Cook time: 6 minutes

FOR THE ASPARAGUS

2 tablespoons avocado oil

1 pound frozen precut asparagus spears

½ teaspoon salt

½ teaspoon freshly ground black pepper

FOR THE SAUCE

1 avocado

¼ cup fresh cilantro leaves

⅔ cup water

Juice of ½ lemon or 1 tablespoon bottled lemon juice

1 peeled garlic clove

¼ teaspoon salt

High in fiber and folate as well as vitamins A, C, E, and K, sautéed asparagus is a great go-to side dish. The nutrient-dense spears can be taken in a variety of directions, but there's just something about sautéing. The tips get a little crispy, and the seasonings hitting the hot oil create a light coating on each spear. As a bonus, the luscious sauce adds a creamy element that features bright acidic bursts.

TO MAKE THE ASPARAGUS

1. In a large skillet, heat the oil over medium-high heat.

2. Microwave the asparagus for 1 minute or until thawed.

3. Add the asparagus, salt, and pepper to the skillet. Sauté for 6 minutes over medium-high heat or until browned on the exterior and tender on the inside. Turn occasionally for even cooking. Remove from the heat.

continued...

ASPARAGUS WITH CREAMY AVOCADO SAUCE *continued*

TO MAKE THE SAUCE

4. In a food processor (or electric food chopper or immersion blender), combine the avocado, cilantro, water, lemon juice, garlic, and salt and process until smooth.

5. Drizzle the asparagus with the sauce and serve.

Tip: Using frozen veggies can ensure that you are maximizing the micronutrients you are getting from them. This is due to the fact that the vegetables are harvested and then flash frozen, which seals in all the vitamins and minerals. You can substitute fresh veggies if you prefer, but frozen works just as well and cuts down on prep time.

Per serving: Calories: 157; Total fat: 13g; Total carbs: 9g; Fiber: 3g; Sugar: 3g; Protein: 4g; Sodium: 451mg

BROCCOLI WITH PINE NUTS AND POMEGRANATE SEEDS

FIVE INGREDIENTS OR LESS, VEGAN

Serves 4
Prep time: 2 minutes
Cook time: 7 minutes

1 pound frozen broccoli florets

2 tablespoons avocado oil

½ teaspoon salt

¼ teaspoon freshly ground black pepper

2 tablespoons pine nuts

½ cup prepackaged pomegranate seeds

Juice of ½ lemon or 1 tablespoon bottled lemon juice

Sautéed broccoli with pine nuts and pomegranate seeds is a refined side dish that is as versatile as it is delicious. Whether it's chicken, beef, or a vegan source of protein, this vegetable dish will complement your entrée beautifully. The broccoli develops flavorful browned bits as it cooks, the pine nuts bring a satisfying crunch, and the pomegranate seeds offer their signature sweet-tart balance.

1. Microwave the broccoli for 1 minute or until thawed.

2. In a large skillet, heat the oil over medium-high heat.

3. Add the broccoli, salt, and pepper. Sauté for 6 minutes while stirring occasionally. Set aside in a serving bowl.

4. Meanwhile, toast the pine nuts in a dry pan over medium-low heat for 2 minutes or until lightly toasted and fragrant.

5. Add the pine nuts and pomegranate seeds to the broccoli. Drizzle with lemon juice, toss, and serve.

Tip: Substitute pine nuts with almonds, pistachios, or pecans if you have them on hand. You can, of course, use fresh broccoli in this recipe if you have the time to wash and cut it.

Per serving: Calories: 153; Total fat: 10g; Total carbs: 11g; Fiber: 4g; Sugar: 6g; Protein: 3g; Sodium: 329mg

CAULIFLOWER RICE SUSHI SALAD

**MAKE-AHEAD,
VEGETARIAN**

Serves 4
Prep time: 7 minutes
Cook time: 3 minutes

FOR THE SALAD

1 tablespoon avocado oil

12 ounces frozen cauliflower
rice, thawed

1 cucumber, diced

2 green onions, thinly sliced

1 avocado, diced

1 or 2 nori sheets, thinly sliced

FOR THE DRESSING

2 tablespoons avocado oil

Juice of 1 lime or
2 tablespoons bottled
lime juice

2 tablespoons tamari or
reduced-sodium soy sauce

1 teaspoon wasabi powder

1 teaspoon honey

Freshly ground black pepper

This recipe combines the key elements of your favorite sushi roll minus the fuss and fish. It includes avocado, cucumber, mildly sweet-sour rice, salty nori, and pungent wasabi, and the umami taste that only fermented soy offers. Frozen riced cauliflower makes this salad veggie-based, low-carb, and super easy to put together.

TO MAKE THE SALAD

1. In a skillet, heat the oil over medium heat.

2. Once the oil is hot, add the cauliflower rice to the skillet. Sauté for 3 minutes.

3. In a bowl, combine the cauliflower rice with the cucumber and green onions.

TO MAKE THE DRESSING

4. In a small bowl, whisk together the oil, lime juice, tamari, wasabi, honey, and pepper (to taste).

5. Pour the dressing over the cauliflower rice, cucumber, and green onions. Toss to coat.

6. Plate, then top with avocado and sliced nori.

Tip: The salad can be eaten immediately but is best served cooled. If you want to include fish, a quickly seared and sliced sushi-grade tuna can be added on top.

....

Per serving: Calories: 195; Total fat: 16g; Total carbs: 13g;
Fiber: 6g; Sugar: 5g; Protein: 4g; Sodium: 528mg

SPINACH SALAD WITH TUNA AND SOFT-BOILED EGG

MAKE-AHEAD

Serves 1
Prep time: 5 minutes
Cook time: 6 minutes

1 large egg, chilled

1½ tablespoons extra-virgin olive oil

Juice of ½ lemon or 1 tablespoon bottled lemon juice

Kosher salt

Freshly ground black pepper

1 (3-ounce) pouch tuna in water

½ small red onion, thinly sliced

⅛ cup pitted Kalamata olives, coarsely chopped

3 cups fresh baby spinach

This salad is super easy to prepare, but has great depth of flavor. Spinach brings its signature bitterness, the red onion has bite, and the olives means your palate gets to experience their distinctively fruity, almost wine-like flavor. The tuna and egg add lean protein to keep you full.

1. In a saucepan, bring 1 inch of water to a boil.

2. Gently place the egg into the saucepan, cover, and cook for 6 minutes.

3. Remove the egg from the saucepan with a slotted spoon and run under cold water. Peel and cut it in half.

4. In a medium bowl, whisk together the oil and lemon juice. Season to taste with salt and pepper.

5. Add the tuna, onion, and olives and toss.

6. Serve over the spinach, top with the egg, and enjoy.

Tip: Soft-boiled eggs can be made up to 3 days in advance. Those who aren't fond of soft-boiled eggs can substitute a hard-boiled egg, cooked for 4 more minutes. For a vegetarian option, replace the egg with ¼ cup of diced tofu and the tuna with ¼ cup of canned chickpeas.

· · · · · · · · · · · · · · · · ·

Per serving: Calories: 391; Total fat: 29g; Total carbs: 9g; Fiber: 3g; Sugar: 3g; Protein: 27g; Sodium: 694mg

SHREDDED BRUSSELS SPROUT SALAD

MAKE-AHEAD, ONE-POT, VEGAN

Serves 4

Prep time: 20 minutes

3 tablespoons extra-virgin olive oil

Juice of 1 lemon or 2 tablespoons bottled lemon juice

1 small shallot, finely chopped

1 tablespoon Dijon mustard

1 garlic clove, minced

1 teaspoon salt, plus more for seasoning

1 (14-ounce) bag Brussels sprouts, shaved

½ cup toasted pine nuts

Freshly ground black pepper

This is definitely a "think outside the box" type of salad, showcasing the crunch of these mini-cabbages as a lettuce substitute. The fresh taste of a lemon vinaigrette is the perfect complement to the bitterness of the raw Brussels sprouts. Kaempferol, a bioflavonoid found in Brussels sprouts, has been shown to have anti-inflammatory properties.

1. In a serving bowl, whisk together the oil, lemon juice, shallot, mustard, garlic, and 1 teaspoon of salt.

2. Add the Brussels sprouts to the bowl and toss. Let them sit for 20 minutes to wilt.

3. Add the pine nuts, season with salt and pepper, and serve.

Tip: The beauty of this dish is that you can make it ahead of time, including mixing in the dressing—no soggy lettuce here! It will last in the refrigerator for 2 days. In a pinch, you can use shredded green cabbage as a substitute for the Brussels sprouts.

Per serving: Calories: 255; Total fat: 22g; Total carbs: 14g; Fiber: 5g; Sugar: 4g; Protein: 6g; Sodium: 704mg

ARUGULA AND FIG SALAD

FIVE INGREDIENTS OR LESS, VEGAN

Serves 4
Prep time: 5 minutes
Cook time: 2 minutes

FOR THE SALAD

5 ounces baby arugula, prewashed

½ cup diced dried or fresh mission figs

¼ cup unsalted, shelled sunflower seeds

¼ cup dry toasted, unsalted slivered almonds

FOR THE BALSAMIC REDUCTION

½ cup balsamic vinegar

Kosher salt

Freshly ground black pepper

Arugula, figs, and a balsamic reduction rich in antioxidants are all you need to make a delicious salad, but this recipe takes it a bit further with the addition of sunflower seeds and almonds. Along with crunch, sunflower seeds add linoleic fatty acids, vitamin E, magnesium, and protein. The almonds have omega-3 fatty acids that help with pain control, as well as essential minerals like calcium, magnesium, and zinc.

TO MAKE THE SALAD

1. In a serving bowl, toss the arugula, figs, sunflower seeds, and almonds.

TO MAKE THE BALSAMIC REDUCTION

2. In a microwave-safe container, microwave the vinegar in 30-second intervals until thick and syrupy, usually 2 to 3 minutes. Season to taste with salt and pepper.

3. Drizzle the vinegar over the salad and serve.

Tip: Arugula can be swapped with a 6-ounce bag of baby spinach or any leafy green you prefer. You can also make the balsamic reduction in a pot on the stove, but the microwave is a faster and easier option.

·················

Per serving: Calories: 139; Total fat: 8g; Total carbs: 14g; Fiber: 3g; Sugar: 10g; Protein: 4g; Sodium: 17mg

SWISS CHARD WITH CHICKPEAS AND ALLSPICE

FIVE INGREDIENTS OR LESS, FREEZER-FRIENDLY, MAKE-AHEAD, VEGAN

Serves 4

Prep time: 7 minutes

Cook time: 10 minutes

2 large bunches Swiss chard, (about 2 pounds)

1½ tablespoons extra-virgin olive oil

1 (15-ounce) can chickpeas, drained and rinsed

½ teaspoon kosher salt

¼ teaspoon garlic powder

¼ teaspoon ground allspice

¼ teaspoon freshly ground black pepper

2 tablespoons water

Swiss chard is a nutritional powerhouse packed with a long list of vitamins and minerals like vitamins A, C, and K, as well as magnesium (for decreasing nerve pain) and manganese. Chickpeas are rich in fiber, polyunsaturated fatty acids, magnesium, and vitamin E. The benefits from both of these plant-based foods combined with their fantastic flavor creates the ultimate side that will pair well with anything, from baked tofu steaks to your favorite fish dish.

1. Wash the chard leaves and stems in a basin of cold water. Gently lift the chard out of the basin, so any grit remains in the water. Rinse with fresh water and shake off any excess moisture before removing the stems from the leaves.

2. Keeping the stems and leaves separate, coarsely chop both.

3. In a large skillet, heat the oil over medium-high heat, then add the chard stems and chickpeas. Season with the salt, garlic powder, allspice, and pepper.

4. Cook for 5 minutes while stirring occasionally. Add the chard leaves in handfuls, stirring to combine.

5. Add the water, cover, and let cook for 4 more minutes before serving. The chard should be tender.

Tip: Easily remove the stems by folding each leaf in half lengthwise. Then use a sharp knife to cut along the edge of the rib.

Per serving: Calories: 182; Total fat: 7g; Total carbs: 24g; Fiber: 8g; Sugar: 5g; Protein: 9g; Sodium: 919mg

KALE SALAD WITH NUTRITIONAL YEAST

FIVE INGREDIENTS OR LESS, MAKE-AHEAD, ONE-POT, VEGAN

Serves 4

Prep time: 5 minutes

4 cups fresh chopped kale

¼ cup extra-virgin olive oil

Pinch salt

¼ cup nutritional yeast

Juice of ½ lemon or 1 tablespoon bottled lemon juice

This hearty, chewy kale salad is such a favorite in my house! Nutritional yeast is loaded with B vitamins, important for energy production and fighting off fatigue. Don't skimp on massaging the kale; this is an important part of breaking down the cell walls and making the kale softer and more palatable. A big part of digestion is chewing food properly, so be sure to chew until the kale is fully broken down. This can help prevent gastrointestinal distress for those that have difficulty with high-fiber foods.

1. Put the kale in a gallon-size resealable bag. Drizzle with the oil, salt, yeast, and lemon juice.

2. Squeeze out any excess air, then seal the bag well. With your hands, knead the kale inside the bag for 2 to 3 minutes until it is wilted.

3. Transfer to bowls and serve.

Tip: If kneading causes you pain, use a rolling pin over the bag to help massage the kale.

....

Per serving: Calories: 148; Total fat: 14g; Total carbs: 3g; Fiber: 2g; Sugar: <1g; Protein: 4g; Sodium: 22mg

ROASTED CHICKPEA SALAD

MAKE-AHEAD, VEGAN

Serves 4
*Prep time: **5 minutes***
*Cook time: **10 minutes***

FOR THE SALAD

2 (15-ounce) cans chickpeas, drained and rinsed

2 tablespoons extra-virgin olive oil

1 teaspoon salt

½ teaspoon freshly ground black pepper

¼ teaspoon garlic powder

2 cups diced cucumber

1 avocado, diced

½ cup chopped fresh flat-leaf parsley

FOR THE VINAIGRETTE

Juice of 1 lime or 2 tablespoons bottled lime juice

2 tablespoons extra-virgin olive oil

The roasted chickpeas are nice and crispy, with a more complex flavor. The warmth elevates the cucumbers from cool to refreshing. The addition of fresh parsley brightens everything up!

TO MAKE THE SALAD

1. Preheat the oven to 425°F and line a baking sheet with parchment paper.

2. Pat the chickpeas dry, then transfer them to the prepared baking sheet.

3. Drizzle the chickpeas with the oil and season with the salt, pepper, and garlic powder. Toss to combine, then spread in an even layer.

4. Roast for 10 minutes. Let cool for 5 minutes.

5. Meanwhile, put the cucumber, avocado, and parsley in a serving bowl.

6. When cooled, transfer the roasted chickpeas to the bowl with the cucumber mixture.

TO MAKE THE VINAIGRETTE

7. In a small bowl, combine the lime juice and oil. Drizzle the dressing over the salad, toss, and serve.

Tip: Roast an extra can or two of chickpeas to use at a later time. They can be refrigerated in an airtight container for up to 1 week.

....

Per serving: Calories: 349; Total fat: 19g; Total carbs: 37g; Fiber: 12g; Sugar: 7g; Protein: 11g; Sodium: 880mg

BEAN TACO SALAD

MAKE-AHEAD, VEGAN

Serves 4

Prep time: 5 minutes

FOR THE SALAD

2 (15-ounce) cans black beans, drained and rinsed

1 avocado, diced

1 (6-ounce) bag salad greens

½ red onion, chopped

¼ cup sliced black olives

FOR THE DRESSING

2 tablespoons avocado oil

Juice of 1 lime or 2 tablespoons bottled lime juice

1 teaspoon ground cumin

⅛ teaspoon garlic powder

⅛ teaspoon salt

This bean taco salad is light, bright, fresh, and hearty. Black beans are an obvious choice, since they're nutrient dense and oh-so-filling. Best of all, they have a mild flavor that plays well with others, along with great mouthfeel. Those delectable characteristics combined with the healthy fat in avocados, crisp lettuce, and antioxidant-rich red onion yield a truly nourishing salad.

TO MAKE THE SALAD

1. In a large salad bowl, combine the beans, avocado, greens, red onion, and olives.

TO MAKE THE DRESSING

2. In a small bowl, whisk together the oil, lime juice, cumin, garlic powder, and salt. Drizzle over the salad and toss.

3. Serve immediately or cover with plastic and chill in the refrigerator to enjoy later.

Tip: Pinto beans are a great substitute for black beans if you don't have them on hand. This salad can be made up to 3 hours in advance.

Per serving: Calories: 355; Total fat: 14g; Total carbs: 47g; Fiber: 20g; Sugar: 1g; Protein: 14g; Sodium: 175mg

CUMIN-SPICED SAUTÉED CABBAGE

**FIVE INGREDIENTS OR
LESS, MAKE-AHEAD,
ONE-POT, VEGAN**

Serves 4
Prep time: 2 minutes
Cook time: 8 minutes

1 tablespoon extra-virgin olive
  oil or avocado oil

1 garlic clove, grated

½ teaspoon ground cumin

3 (10-ounce) bags
  shredded cabbage

¼ teaspoon kosher salt

Juice of ½ lemon or
  1 tablespoon bottled
  lemon juice

Freshly ground black pepper

¼ teaspoon grated lemon zest

*Tender and caramelized with hints of garlic
throughout, this sautéed cabbage is just the thing
to take your favorite entrée to the next level. Garlic
is joined by smoky cumin for depth of flavor and
anti-inflammatory properties along with a hint of
lemon juice, which enhances the natural flavor of the
leafy greens while keeping this side light and bright.*

1. In a large saucepan, heat the oil over medium heat.

2. Add the garlic and cumin. Cook, while stirring, for
    30 seconds.

3. Add the cabbage and salt. Continue to stir for
    another 30 seconds to incorporate everything.

4. Cook for 7 minutes. Stir occasionally or until the
    cabbage is wilted and slightly brown.

5. Remove the pan from the heat and pour in the
    lemon juice. Toss.

6. Season to taste with salt and pepper, then garnish
    with lemon zest.

Tip: To ensure the cabbage retains some bite, do not exceed the
recommended cook time. Avoiding overcooking also prevents
the unpleasant smell that cooked cabbage can develop.

....

Per serving: Calories: 94; Total fat: 3g; Total carbs: 13g; Fiber: 6g;
Sugar: 6g; Protein: 3g; Sodium: 194mg

*Maple-Orange Grilled Tempeh
with Sweet Potato* ▸ *page 48*

Chapter 4

MEATLESS MAINS

ROASTED TOFU SHAWARMA WITH TURMERIC CAULIFLOWER RICE

VEGAN

Serves 4
Prep time: 5 minutes
Cook time: 20 minutes

1 (16-ounce) block
  extra-firm tofu

5 tablespoons extra-virgin
  olive oil, divided

1 tablespoon Shawarma
  Seasoning (page 118)

1 yellow onion, diced

1 teaspoon ground turmeric

¼ teaspoon garlic powder

12 ounces frozen cauliflower
  rice, thawed

Salt

Freshly ground black pepper

1 Persian cucumber, halved
  lengthwise and diced

1 cup fresh baby spinach

This tofu shawarma is warm, complex, and a touch tangy—and delivers a series of bold flavors when paired with turmeric cauliflower rice. The double dose of the turmeric, both in the cauliflower rice and the shawarma seasoning, makes sure you get more than your daily dose of this anti-inflammatory spice. This complete meal can be served alone or with a side of tzatziki for extra tang.

1. Preheat the oven to 425°F and line a baking sheet with parchment paper.

2. Firmly squeeze the tofu over a bowl to expel as much water as possible, then cut it into 1-inch pieces.

3. Drizzle the tofu with 4 tablespoons of oil, then season with the spice blend. Toss, then arrange in an even layer on the baking sheet.

4. Roast for 20 minutes or until golden, flipping halfway through.

5. During the last 10 minutes of cook time, heat the remaining 1 tablespoon of oil in a large skillet over medium heat.

6. Sauté the onion for 5 minutes, or until softened and fragrant.

7. Add the turmeric, garlic powder, and cauliflower rice. Cook, stirring occasionally, for 5 minutes. Season to taste with salt and pepper.

8. To serve, divide the cauliflower rice onto plates and top with the cucumbers, spinach, and tofu.

Tip: If you cannot find extra-firm tofu, firm tofu will work well in this recipe, too. For added chewiness, you can substitute tempeh for tofu. If squeezing the tofu is too difficult, put a paper towel or clean dish towel over the tofu block, then rest a heavy pan on top for 5 minutes to squeeze out the liquid.

....

Per serving: Calories: 312; Total fat: 23g; Total carbs: 13g; Fiber: 5g; Sugar: 3g; Protein: 15g; Sodium: 37mg

MAPLE-ORANGE GRILLED TEMPEH WITH SWEET POTATO

VEGAN

Serves 1
Prep time: 7 minutes
Cook time: 14 minutes

3 ounces tempeh

Kosher salt

Freshly ground black pepper

1 tablespoon maple syrup

1 teaspoon orange juice

1/2 teaspoon avocado oil

1/8 teaspoon ground ginger

1 medium sweet potato

1/2 tablespoon coconut oil

1/8 teaspoon ground cinnamon

1/8 teaspoon grated orange zest

Maple syrup and orange contrast with the earthy flavor of the tempeh beautifully, and it only gets better after a few minutes on the grill. All that flavor together with the cinnamon and orange zest-infused mashed sweet potatoes keep the flavor bright and delightful. This is surely a vegan meal worth boasting about.

1. Bring a medium pot of water to a simmer.

2. Cut the tempeh diagonally into triangles, then blanch in the simmering water for 5 minutes.

3. Pat the tempeh dry, then generously season it with salt and pepper.

4. In a small bowl, combine the maple syrup, orange juice, avocado oil, and ginger. Brush the tempeh with this mixture.

5. Heat a nonstick grill pan over medium-high heat. Grill the tempeh for 3 minutes per side or until the light glaze has caramelized.

6. Meanwhile, pierce the potato several times and wrap it in a damp paper towel. Microwave for 5 to 8 minutes, until you can easily stick a fork through it.

7. Halve the potato in half lengthwise and scoop the flesh into a bowl, discarding the skin.

....

8. Mash the sweet potato with the coconut oil, cinnamon, and orange zest. Serve with the tempeh.

Tip: Brush the tempeh with the glaze and let it sit for 30 minutes in the refrigerator or overnight for even more flavor.

....

Per serving: Calories: 439; Total fat: 17g; Total carbs: 52g; Fiber: 14g; Sugar: 18g; Protein: 21g; Sodium: 74mg

GLUTEN-FREE PARSLEY-PESTO PASTA WITH KALAMATA OLIVES

VEGAN

Serves 4
Prep time: 10 minutes
Cook time: 10 minutes

Kosher salt

2 cups packed fresh basil

1 cup packed fresh
  flat-leaf parsley

½ cup almonds

3 garlic cloves, peeled

1 teaspoon grated lemon zest

Juice of ½ lemon or
  1 tablespoon bottled
  lemon juice

¾ cup extra-virgin olive oil,
  plus more if needed

Freshly ground black pepper

1 pound gluten-free pasta
  of choice

½ cup chopped
  Kalamata olives

Basil, parsley, almonds, lemon, and a few other additions combine to create a light and bright pesto sauce that takes gluten-free pasta to new heights. When the aroma hits your nose, the freshness takes over your palate and the fruity, briny flavor from the olives delivers the perfect finish.

1. Bring a large pot of water to a boil. Salt generously once boiling.

2. In a food processor or blender, combine the basil, parsley, almonds, garlic, lemon zest, and lemon juice. Pulse until combined.

3. Add the oil and blend until the pesto is smooth.

4. Season the pesto with salt and pepper, then set aside.

5. Add the pasta to the boiling water and cook according to the package instructions. Drain.

6. Spoon as much or as little of the pesto as you'd like over the pasta. Top with the olives and serve.

Tip: Pour enough oil on the top of the leftover pesto to completely cover it before refrigerating it.

....

Per serving: Calories: 887; Total fat: 53g; Total carbs: 93g; Fiber: 6g; Sugar: 1g; Protein: 14g; Sodium: 326mg

BAKED HEMP-SEED FALAFEL WITH CURRY-YOGURT SAUCE

FREEZER-FRIENDLY, MAKE-AHEAD, VEGAN

Serves 4

Prep time: 10 minutes

Cook time: 20 minutes

FOR THE FALAFEL

1 cup canned chickpeas, drained and rinsed

½ cup fresh flat-leaf parsley

¼ cup chopped fresh mint

2 garlic cloves, peeled

⅓ cup hemp seeds (hemp hearts)

½ yellow onion, chopped

2 heaping tablespoons ground flaxseed meal

2 teaspoons ground cumin

1 teaspoon kosher salt

½ teaspoon freshly ground black pepper

½ teaspoon dried coriander

¼ teaspoon curry powder

2 tablespoons extra-virgin olive oil

Arugula, for serving

FOR THE CURRY-YOGURT SAUCE

1 cup unsweetened coconut yogurt

1½ teaspoons curry powder

Juice of ½ lime or 1 tablespoon bottled lime juice

Loaded with fiber, fresh herbs, and healthy fat, baked hemp-seed falafels make for an incredible meatless meal. Their complex flavor profile paired with the creamy, cool contrast of the yogurt-based sauce are sure to leave the palate wanting more. The curry in this recipe shines as a pain reliever, so it is used in both the falafel and the dipping sauce. One study, published in the European Review for Medical and Pharmacological Sciences *(2017), found that curcumin, the active ingredient in curry, was as effective in relieving pain in rugby players as traditional pain-relieving drugs.*

TO MAKE THE FALAFEL

1. Preheat the oven to 400°F. Line a baking sheet with parchment paper.

2. In the bowl of a food processor, combine the chickpeas, parsley, mint, and garlic.

3. Add the hemp seeds, onion, flaxseed, cumin, salt, pepper, coriander, and curry powder to the food processor. Process until mostly smooth with some remaining lumps.

4. Scoop the falafel mixture from the food processor in 2-tablespoon portions. Roll into balls and place onto the prepared baking sheet. Brush with the oil.

continued...

BAKED HEMP-SEED FALAFEL WITH CURRY-YOGURT SAUCE *continued*

5. Bake for 20 minutes, turning halfway through.

6. Serve on a bed of arugula.

TO MAKE THE CURRY-YOGURT SAUCE

7. In a small bowl, whisk together the yogurt, curry powder, and lime juice, then refrigerate while the falafel is baking.

8. Drizzle the dressing over the bed of arugula with falafel.

Tip: If the falafel mixture is too sticky to handle, add an extra teaspoon of flaxseed meal.

Per serving: Calories: 271; Total fat: 18g; Total carbs: 19g; Fiber: 6g; Sugar: 3g; Protein: 9g; Sodium: 614mg

SAUTÉED CABBAGE WITH WALNUTS

VEGAN

Serves 4
Prep time: 7 minutes
Cook time: 15 minutes

FOR THE WALNUT "MEAT"

2 cups raw walnuts

1 tablespoon low-sodium
    soy sauce

1/4 teaspoon freshly ground
    black pepper

FOR THE CABBAGE

1 tablespoon extra-virgin olive
    oil or avocado oil

1/2 yellow onion,
    finely chopped

2 garlic cloves, minced

1/2 teaspoon ground cumin

1/4 teaspoon ground ginger

3 (10-ounce) bags
    shredded cabbage

Juice of 1/2 lemon or
    1 tablespoon bottled
    lemon juice

1/4 teaspoon kosher salt

Freshly ground black pepper

This sautéed cabbage is full of flavor. The walnut "meat" serves as a tasty, crunchy addition to the meal. The cabbage can also reduce swelling and inflammatory markers. This star should definitely be a staple in any fibro warrior's meal plan.

TO MAKE THE WALNUT "MEAT"

1. In a food processor, combine the walnuts, soy sauce, and pepper. Pulse until coarse and crumbly.

TO MAKE THE CABBAGE

2. In a large skillet, heat the oil over medium heat.

3. Sauté the onion for 5 minutes.

4. Add the garlic and cook for another minute before adding the cumin and ginger. Cook for 30 seconds.

5. Toss in the cabbage. Cook for 7 minutes while stirring occasionally, until the cabbage is wilted and slightly browned.

6. Add the walnut "meat" and continue to cook, stirring, for 2 minutes or until warmed through.

7. Remove from the heat and pour in the lemon juice. Toss and season with salt and pepper to taste.

Tip: Swap the soy sauce for tamari if gluten-free, or for coconut aminos if you do not consume soy. Always check the ingredients of soy sauce, as some may have added MSG.

....

Per serving: Calories: 431; Total fat: 36g; Total carbs: 22g; Fiber: 10g; Sugar: 8g; Protein: 11g; Sodium: 339mg

ZUCCHINI NOODLE "ALFREDO" WITH TOASTED PUMPKIN SEEDS

VEGAN

Serves 4
Prep time: 7 minutes
Cook time: 4 minutes

1 cup raw cashews

¾ cup hot water

2 garlic cloves, peeled

½ teaspoon onion powder

1 teaspoon kosher salt

½ teaspoon freshly ground black pepper

1 tablespoon extra-virgin olive oil

32 ounces fresh packaged zucchini noodles, or 5 medium zucchini, spiralized

¼ cup chopped fresh flat-leaf parsley

¼ cup dry roasted, shelled pumpkin seeds

This dairy-free alternative to traditional Alfredo sauce is just as rich and creamy but is made with cashews. The good fats in the nutrient-dense nuts allow them to achieve the ideal consistency for a luscious sauce. All that goodness is served over fresh zucchini noodles, topped with parsley, and finished with toasted pumpkin seeds to create a nourishing plate of food.

1. In a powerful blender or food processor, combine the cashews, water, garlic, onion powder, salt, and pepper. Blend or process until smooth and creamy.

2. In a large skillet, heat the oil over medium heat.

3. Add the zucchini noodles once the oil is hot. Sauté for 3 to 4 minutes or until warmed through.

4. Add the sauce to the skillet and toss again.

5. Top with parsley and pumpkin seeds before serving.

Tip: Soak the cashews in water overnight if you do not have a powerful food processor or blender.

....

Per serving: Calories: 297; Total fat: 21g; Total carbs: 20g; Fiber: 5g; Sugar: 7g; Protein: 11g; Sodium: 611mg

SWEET POTATO TOAST WITH AVOCADO AND SAUERKRAUT

FIVE INGREDIENTS OR LESS, VEGAN

*Serves **2***
*Prep time: **3 minutes***
*Cook time: **12 minutes***

2 sweet potatoes, cut lengthwise into ¼-inch-thick slices

1 avocado, mashed

¼ teaspoon salt

⅓ cup sauerkraut

This bread-free toast will delight your senses with its crunchy, creamy, and tangy layers of goodness. The omega-3 fatty acids from the avocado help decrease pain, while the sauerkraut offers up vitamin C, vitamin K, and probiotics to maintain gut health. For optimal benefit, purchase sauerkraut that is in the refrigerated section. Most canned varieties have been pasteurized and are therefore missing out on the good bacteria this recipe offers.

1. Pop the sweet potato slices into the toaster and toast two to three times on high. If you do not have a toaster, set the oven to broil and broil on an oiled baking sheet for 3 to 6 minutes per side (or until golden brown).

2. Top the sweet potato toasts with mashed avocado and season with salt. Top with sauerkraut and serve.

Tip: You can mash the avocado ahead of time and keep it in the fridge until you're ready to use it. Just mash it, put it in a bowl, and add water on top to cover. When you want to use it, pour off the excess water and give it a quick mix. The avocado will be ready to use and perfectly green.

....

Per serving: Calories: 233; Total fat: 11g; Total carbs: 34g; Fiber: 10g; Sugar: 0g; Protein: 4g; Sodium: 629mg

SUNFLOWER SEED "TUNA" IN LETTUCE CUPS

VEGAN

Serves 4
Prep time: 10 minutes
Cook time: 10 minutes

1½ cups raw sunflower seeds

½ small red onion

4 black olives

2 nori sheets

¾ teaspoon freshly ground
    black pepper, divided

1 tablespoon extra-virgin
    olive oil

1 avocado, halved

Juice of 1 lemon or
    2 tablespoons bottled
    lemon juice

½ teaspoon salt

8 romaine lettuce leaves

1 cucumber, julienned

¼ cup matchstick
    (julienned) carrots

This vegan tuna salad is made with sunflower seeds, black olives, and nori to create a flavor reminiscent of tuna. While the brininess of the black olive and salty nori duo mimics the taste of fish, the avocado brings good fat to the recipe, and it helps achieve the texture that every good "tuna" salad should have.

1. Bring a medium pot of water to a boil.

2. Add the sunflower seeds and let boil for 10 minutes.

3. Drain the sunflower seeds. In a food processor, combine the sunflower seeds, onion, olives, nori, ½ teaspoon of pepper, and oil. Process until ground into small pieces.

4. In a medium bowl, mash the avocado with the lemon juice, salt, and remaining ¼ teaspoon of pepper before adding the sunflower seed mixture. Stir to combine.

5. Divide the sunflower seed "tuna" among the romaine leaves and top with cucumber and carrots. Eat as you would a taco.

Tip: These lettuce boats can be eaten right away or stored as made-ahead components. Try out different types of greens, such as collard greens or endive leaves, for a different flavor.

....

Per serving: Calories: 431; Total fat: 36g; Total carbs: 21g; Fiber: 10g; Sugar: 4g; Protein: 14g; Sodium: 351mg

BROCCOLI WITH VEGAN "CHEDDAR" SAUCE

VEGAN

Serves 3
Prep time: 5 minutes
Cook time: 6 minutes

4 cups frozen broccoli florets

2 cups cashews

2 cups unsweetened cashew
 milk or other nut milk

3 tablespoons
 nutritional yeast

1 teaspoon soy sauce or tamari

½ teaspoon garlic powder

¼ teaspoon freshly ground
 black pepper

Pinch ground nutmeg

Rich and cheesy without the actual cheese, this vegan broccoli and "cheese" is your new go-to recipe when you want comfort food in a pinch. This recipe is made entirely in the microwave, so it is super easy! The sauce is cashew based, with nutritional yeast added to achieve a cheesy taste. Frozen broccoli is used to keep prep time minimal, but fresh broccoli can also be used. Findings published in a 2014 Nutrition Research *article observed a decrease of inflammation and oxidative stress in mice who were fed a diet that included broccoli.*

1. In a microwave-safe bowl, microwave the broccoli florets for about 1 minute to thaw, then cut into smaller pieces.

2. Return to the bowl, cover, and microwave for another 3 to 4 minutes or until warmed through but slightly firm.

3. In a food processor or blender, combine the cashews, milk, yeast, soy sauce, garlic powder, pepper, and nutmeg. Process until smooth. Add more cashew milk 1 tablespoon at a time if needed to achieve the desired consistency.

continued...

BROCCOLI WITH VEGAN "CHEDDAR" SAUCE *continued*

4. Add the sauce to the broccoli, tossing to coat. You may not need all of the sauce.

5. Microwave for another minute to warm the sauce through, and serve.

Tip: Soak cashews in water overnight if you do not have a powerful food processor or blender.

Per serving: Calories: 564; Total fat: 40g; Total carbs: 35g; Fiber: 7g; Sugar: 8g; Protein: 22g; Sodium: 259mg

VEGETARIAN BEEF CRUMBLE WITH CAULIFLOWER MASH

FIVE INGREDIENTS OR LESS, FREEZER-FRIENDLY, MAKE-AHEAD, VEGAN

Serves 2
*Prep time: **7 minutes***
*Cook time: **10 minutes***

1 pound frozen cauliflower

2 garlic cloves, peeled

2 tablespoons extra-virgin olive oil, divided

8 ounces plant-based beef crumbles, thawed

¼ teaspoon dried parsley

⅛ teaspoon dried oregano

¼ teaspoon kosher salt

⅛ teaspoon freshly ground black pepper

This meatless version of beefy mashed potato bowls is filling and flavorful. The cauliflower keeps carbs low while plant-based meat crumbles replaces beef. This dish is nice and garlicky. The crumbles bring a beefiness to the meal along with protein and texture variation.

1. Bring a pot of water to a boil.

2. Add the cauliflower and garlic and cook for 10 minutes or until fork-tender.

3. Drain the cauliflower and garlic, pat dry, and set aside.

4. In a skillet, heat 1 tablespoon of oil over medium-high heat, add the plant-based beef crumbles, and cook for 1 minute while stirring. Set aside.

5. Add the remaining 1 tablespoon of oil and the parsley, oregano, salt, and pepper to the cauliflower and garlic. Mash with a potato masher.

6. Transfer to bowls, add the beef crumbles, and serve.

Tip: Add 1 tablespoon of plant-based milk, plain coconut yogurt, or vegan cream cheese to achieve a creamier consistency. Mashed cauliflower can be stored for up to 3 months in a freezer.

....

Per serving: Calories:364; Total fat: 20g; Total carbs: 18g; Fiber: 7g; Sugar: 5g; Protein: 30g; Sodium: 845mg

PERSIAN BEAN STEW WITH DILL AND PARSLEY

FREEZER-FRIENDLY, MAKE-AHEAD, ONE-POT, VEGAN

Serves 4
Prep time: 5 minutes
Cooking time: 20 minutes

3 tablespoons extra-virgin olive oil

2 onions, diced

2 garlic cloves, minced

2 (15-ounce) cans chickpeas, drained

1 (15-ounce) can cannellini beans, drained

1 (15-ounce) can red kidney beans, drained

1 tablespoon turmeric

9 cups vegetable broth (page 115 for a homemade version)

1 beet, diced

1 pound gluten-free fettuccini noodles

1 teaspoon salt

¼ teaspoon freshly ground black pepper

2 cups chopped fresh dill

3 cups chopped fresh flat-leaf parsley

10 ounces frozen spinach

1 (15-ounce) can lentils, drained and rinsed

Vegan sour cream, for serving

I was first introduced to this dish when my Persian friend made it for me, and I was hooked just from the aroma alone! This hearty melding of flavors truly hits the spot. This version is modified to minimize time while maximizing flavor. The recipe blends the sweetness of fresh dill with the powerful flavors of several nutrient-dense beans and legumes, providing both excellent nutritional and culinary power.

1. In a large pot, heat the oil over medium-high heat.

2. Add the onion and sauté until slightly browned, about 7 minutes. Add the garlic and continue cooking for 1 minute. Remove 1 spoonful of the onion mixture and set it aside for garnish.

3. Add the chickpeas, cannellini beans, kidney beans, turmeric, broth, beet, fettuccini, salt, pepper, dill, parsley, spinach, and lentils. Simmer, covered, on low heat for 20 minutes. Be careful not to let it boil over.

4. Serve warm and garnish with the reserved onion mixture and a little vegan sour cream.

Tip: You can make a large batch and freeze half of this recipe in individual portions to use when you don't feel like cooking. For added flavor, you can also add ½ cup of chopped cilantro.

Per serving: Calories: 1,089; Total fat: 18g; Total carbs: 193g; Fiber: 36g; Sugar: 20g; Protein: 42g; Sodium: 2,609mg

CAULIFLOWER STEAK WITH MUSHROOM GRAVY

VEGAN

Serves 2

Prep time: 10 minutes

Cook time: 20 minutes

FOR THE STEAKS

1 large head cauliflower

1 teaspoon garlic powder

½ teaspoon kosher salt

½ teaspoon freshly ground black pepper

2 tablespoons extra-virgin olive oil

FOR THE GRAVY

1½ tablespoons vegetable oil

½ yellow onion, diced

4 ounces presliced baby bella mushrooms, coarsely chopped

2 tablespoons coconut flour

¾ cup vegetable broth (page 115) or store-bought

1 cup unsweetened almond milk

1 tablespoon low-sodium soy sauce or tamari

¼ teaspoon garlic powder

¼ teaspoon kosher salt

¼ teaspoon freshly ground black pepper

This is an elegant, full-flavored vegan main. For this recipe, fresh cauliflower is needed to yield large steak-like pieces, while baby bellas are recommended for the gravy due to their earthy, meaty taste. Cruciferous vegetables like cauliflower contain sulforaphane, an antioxidant which has been shown to reduce nerve-related pain and inflammation in mice models. Also of note, when comparing cruciferous vegetable extract to Tramadol, a prescription painkiller, a 2017 study published in Food & Function *found that the extract seemed to work as effectively as the drug.*

TO MAKE THE STEAKS

1. Preheat the oven to 450°F. Line a baking sheet with parchment paper.

2. Remove the outer leaves from the cauliflower, trim the stem, and halve lengthwise.

3. Cut into 1½-inch-thick steaks and place them on the prepared baking sheet. Season both sides of each steak with garlic powder, salt, and pepper, then drizzle with the oil.

4. Cover the baking sheet with foil, seal tightly, and bake for 6 minutes. Remove the foil and roast for 7 minutes per side.

continued...

CAULIFLOWER STEAK WITH MUSHROOM GRAVY *continued*

TO MAKE THE GRAVY

5. In a saucepan, heat the oil over medium heat. Sauté the onion and mushrooms for 3 minutes.

6. Whisk in the flour and cook for 1 minute.

7. In a bowl, combine the broth, almond milk, and soy sauce. Add the liquid to the saucepan as you whisk. Season with garlic powder, salt, and pepper.

8. Simmer for 7 minutes. Pour over the steaks and serve.

Tip: Wipe mushrooms with a damp cloth to clean. It's important not to douse mushrooms in water since this can affect their taste and texture.

Per serving: Calories: 403; Total fat: 27g; Total carbs: 34g; Fiber: 12g; Sugar: 11g; Protein: 13g; Sodium: 1,454mg

Roasted Salmon with Lemon and Orange ▸ *page 73*

Chapter 5

🌿

FISH

ROSEMARY AND HONEY OVEN-BAKED SALMON

FIVE INGREDIENTS OR LESS, ONE-POT

Serves 4
Prep time: 3 minutes
Cook time: 15 minutes

4 (6-ounce) boneless, skinless salmon fillets

1 tablespoon honey

2 tablespoons minced fresh rosemary

1 teaspoon salt

½ teaspoon freshly ground black pepper

The piney aroma and sharp flavor of rosemary paired with the sweetness of honey enhance the mild-flavored fish, while baking adds more nuance of flavor. The sugar from the honey caramelizes, resulting in a complexity that deepens the taste of the fish. This recipe works with any good-quality salmon, but make sure to fully thaw the fillets in the refrigerator if frozen.

1. Preheat the oven to 425°F and line a baking sheet with parchment paper.

2. Pat the salmon fillets dry with a paper towel, then transfer them to the baking sheet. Brush with the honey.

3. In a small bowl, combine the rosemary, salt, and pepper. Sprinkle over the top of each fillet.

4. Bake for 15 minutes, or until the fish easily flakes.

5. Remove from the oven and serve with your favorite side.

Tip: Drape salmon fillets over the edge of a bowl to check for pin bones. Often one or two are overlooked. Use tweezers to extract them.

....

Per serving: Calories: 213; Total fat: 7g; Total carbs: 5g; Fiber: <1g; Sugar: 7g; Protein: 33g; Sodium: 845mg

GINGER-SOY AHI TUNA STEAK

FIVE INGREDIENTS OR LESS, ONE-POT

Serves 2
Prep time: 18 minutes
Cook time: 4 minutes

2 (4-ounce) ahi tuna steaks

2 tablespoons soy sauce or tamari

Juice of ½ lime or 1 tablespoon bottled lime juice

1 teaspoon grated ginger

1 tablespoon avocado oil

Ahi tuna is best kept simple. Marinating the firm-flesh fish in soy sauce, lime juice, and ginger plays up its natural flavor, while a quick sear on each side adds a bit of texture. Although ahi tuna is best served rare with its pink flesh on display, it can be cooked to medium or even medium-well. Just avoid overcooking to prevent the fish from becoming tough.

1. In a food-safe resealable bag, combine the steaks, soy sauce, lime juice, and ginger. Seal and move the contents of the bag around to evenly coat the steaks. Let marinate for 15 minutes.

2. When the 15 minutes is almost up, heat a dry, medium nonstick skillet over high heat for about 3 minutes, or until searing hot.

3. Pour the oil into the skillet. Sear the steaks on all sides until the desired doneness is achieved.

4. Transfer the tuna to a cutting board and let rest for 3 minutes.

5. Cut into ½-inch-thick slices and serve.

Tip: For the best result, use ahi tuna steaks that are about 1½ inches thick. Cook for 1 minute per side for rare, 1 minute and 30 seconds for medium, and 1 minute and 45 seconds for medium-well.

Per serving: Calories: 198; Total fat: 7g; Total carbs: 2g; Fiber: <1g; Sugar: 1g; Protein: 29g; Sodium: 927mg

SARDINE SPREAD ON CUCUMBER ROUNDS

FIVE INGREDIENTS OR LESS, MAKE-AHEAD, ONE-POT

Serves 2

Prep time: 3 minutes

6 ounces canned sardines in oil, drained

3 tablespoons mayonnaise

⅓ cup apple cider vinegar

1 cucumber, cut into rounds

This is an unusual choice of fish for most people, but don't knock it until you've tried it! Most people are pleasantly surprised by the mild flavor of sardines, which is not fishy at all. Sardines are high in vitamin D as well as omega-3 fatty acids, the kind of fat that can help reduce inflammation. Sardines are also known to be low in mercury, which is an added bonus for brain health.

1. In a bowl, mash together the sardines, mayonnaise, and vinegar.

2. Spoon the sardine spread onto each cucumber round and serve.

Tip: Sub out cucumbers with any vegetable of your choice, such as romaine lettuce or endive leaf "boats," carrot rounds, or jicama rounds. You can also add fresh herbs or freshly ground black pepper on top for more flavor.

Per serving: Calories: 342; Total fat: 25g; Total carbs: 4g; Fiber: 1g; Sugar: 2g; Protein: 22g; Sodium: 396mg

GRILLED MACKEREL FILLET WITH BLACK-EYED PEA SALAD

......

MAKE-AHEAD

Serves 2

Prep time: 10 minutes

Cook time: 8 minutes

FOR THE MACKEREL

2 fresh or defrosted
mackerel fillets

1 teaspoon extra-virgin
olive oil

Kosher salt

Freshly ground black pepper

FOR THE SALAD

2 tablespoons extra-virgin
olive oil

Juice of 1 lime or
2 tablespoons bottled
lime juice

1 (15-ounce) can black-eyed
peas, drained and rinsed

1/2 cup chopped fresh
flat-leaf parsley

1/2 cup chopped fresh cilantro

3 green onions, cut diagonally

1 celery stalk, finely diced

Kosher salt

Freshly ground black pepper

Mackerel is inexpensive and nutritious, and its bolder taste pairs beautifully with the freshness of the salad. As a plus, it is rich in healthy omega-3 fatty acids, coenzyme Q10, and antioxidants, which help prevent inflammatory responses.

TO MAKE THE MACKEREL

1. Prepare a grill or grill pan for high-heat cooking.

2. Brush the fish with oil and lightly season both sides with salt and pepper.

3. Grill for 4 minutes per side or until just cooked through.

4. Remove from the grill and let rest for 2 minutes.

TO MAKE THE SALAD

5. In a medium bowl, whisk together the oil and lime juice.

6. Add the black-eyed peas, parsley, cilantro, green onions, celery, and salt and pepper to taste. Toss to combine.

7. Plate the fish and serve with the salad.

Tip: The salad can be served immediately but tastes better when chilled for at least an hour.

....

Per serving: Calories: 557; Total fat: 34g; Total carbs: 33g; Fiber: 9g; Sugar: 3g; Protein: 33g; Sodium: 184mg

PAN-SEARED TROUT WITH TZATZIKI

**FIVE INGREDIENTS
OR LESS**

Serves 4
Prep time: 7 minutes
Cook time: 8 minutes

4 (4-ounce) fresh or frozen
trout fillets, skin on

Kosher salt

Freshly ground black pepper

2 tablespoons extra-virgin
olive oil

Juice of ½ lemon or
1 tablespoon bottled
lemon juice

Dairy-Free Tzatziki (page 111)

Pan-seared trout has a great exterior texture and a delicate mild taste, which gets even better when accompanied by tzatziki. The tzatziki adds a creamy element with some healthy fat. Trout, a freshwater fish, is a relative of salmon and has a low mercury level and a high omega-3 fatty acid content; this helps reduce inflammation in the body.

1. Pat each fillet dry and generously season both sides with salt and pepper.

2. In a large nonstick skillet, heat the oil over medium-high heat.

3. Once the oil is hot, place the trout fillets into the skillet, skin-side down. Cook for 5 minutes.

4. Carefully flip and cook for another 3 minutes or until the fish easily flakes with a fork.

5. Pour the lemon juice into the hot skillet and use a spoon to baste each fillet.

6. Remove from the pan. Serve with the tzatziki.

Tip: Buying fish with the skin on helps keep the fillet from falling apart as it cooks. If you prefer skinless, it is best to bake the fish in a covered dish at 350°F in the oven for 20 to 25 minutes.

....

Per serving: Calories: 215; Total fat: 13g; Total carbs: <1g; Fiber: 0g; Sugar: <1g; Protein: 24g; Sodium: 41mg

TUNA BURGERS ON A BED OF ARUGULA

MAKE-AHEAD

Serves 4

Prep time: 10 minutes

Cook time: 10 minutes

1 (24 ounce) can chunk light tuna, drained

1 large egg, lightly beaten

½ cup unsweetened coconut or Greek yogurt, divided

⅓ cup coconut or almond flour

1 teaspoon cumin

1 teaspoon garlic powder

¼ teaspoon onion powder

2 tablespoons extra-virgin olive oil, divided

Kosher salt

Freshly ground black pepper

3 cups baby arugula

Lime wedges, for serving

These protein-packed tuna burgers are meaty, filling, and perfectly seasoned, and the arugula adds a peppery bite. An egg, your favorite unsweetened yogurt, and a few other additions are all you need to turn a can of tuna into a healthy low carb meal, giving you ample protein to maintain muscles. The arugula is jam-packed with isothiocyanates, which aid the body in reducing overall inflammation.

1. In a bowl, combine the tuna, egg, ¼ cup of coconut yogurt, the flour, cumin, garlic powder, onion powder, and 1 tablespoon of oil until well mixed.

2. Form into four equal-sized patties.

3. In a large skillet, heat the remaining 1 tablespoon of oil over medium-high heat.

4. Season both sides with salt and pepper.

5. Cook for 5 minutes per side or until golden brown.

6. Serve over a bed of arugula with ¼ cup of yogurt and lime wedges.

Tip: Tuna burgers can be wrapped in plastic, and refrigerated for up to 2 days. Add a bit more flour if the mixture does not form well into patties. It is best to purchase skipjack or chunk light canned tuna because albacore tuna has a higher mercury content.

....

Per serving: Calories: 251; Total fat: 13g; Total carbs: 8g; Fiber: 4g; Sugar: 1g; Protein: 28g; Sodium: 451mg

WHITE WINE HALIBUT WITH ARTICHOKE HEARTS

ONE-POT

Serves 2

*Prep time: **5 minutes***

*Cook time: **15 minutes***

1 tablespoon extra-virgin
   olive oil

2 (6-ounce) halibut fillets

Salt

Freshly ground black pepper

⅓ cup dry white wine

1 (6-ounce) jar small artichoke
   hearts, drained

1 yellow onion, chopped

2 garlic cloves, minced

Juice of ½ lemon or
   1 tablespoon bottled
   lemon juice

Seared halibut has a nice crust on the exterior. When the fish is finished in the oven, the mild, sweet-tasting flesh works well with the nutty and subtly sweet taste of artichoke hearts. The white wine enhances the flavor of both the artichokes and the fish.

1. Preheat the oven to 425°F.

2. In an oven-safe skillet, heat the oil over medium-high heat.

3. Generously season both sides of each fillet with salt and pepper. Place the fish in the pan and sear for 3 minutes. Flip the fish and sear for an additional 2 minutes.

4. Pour in the wine and let simmer for 2 minutes. Toss in the artichoke hearts, chopped onion, and garlic. Simmer for another 2 minutes.

5. Put the skillet into the oven and bake for 5 minutes.

6. Remove from the oven, drizzle with lemon juice, plate, and serve.

Tip: For best results, use a wine that you enjoy drinking! You can transfer the fillets first to an oven-safe dish, adding the sauce and artichokes from the pan if you don't have an oven-safe pan.

Per serving: Calories: 375; Total fat: 11g; Total carbs: 13g; Fiber: 4g; Sugar: 3g; Protein: 46g; Sodium: 193mg

ROASTED SALMON WITH LEMON AND ORANGE

FIVE INGREDIENTS OR LESS, ONE-POT

Serves 4
Prep time: 5 minutes
Cook time: 10 minutes

Grated lemon zest and 4 fresh lemon slices

Grated orange zest and 4 fresh orange slices

4 (6- to 8-ounce) skinless salmon fillets

Pinch kosher salt

Freshly ground black pepper

1 tablespoon extra-virgin olive oil

⅔ cup white wine

This citrusy salmon dish is always a crowd-pleaser. The tender flesh is very nicely complemented by the white wine and citrus combination. This recipe takes very little time to put together, but the presentation on sliced fruit elevates it to a great entertaining dish sure to garner compliments for the chef! Salmon is high in omega-3 fatty acids, which can help alleviate inflammation.

1. Preheat the oven to 375°F.

2. In a 9-by-13-inch baking dish, place one lemon slice and one orange slice side by side, making a "bed" for each piece of salmon. Repeat with the rest of the slices.

3. Top each "bed" with a piece of salmon and sprinkle with salt and pepper. Drizzle the oil on top.

4. Pour the wine over the salmon, then sprinkle the lemon and orange zest on each piece. Bake for 8 to 10 minutes and serve.

Tip: You can also use salmon fillets with the skin on if that is the only kind available. This dish can be assembled in the morning and cooked later in the day, pouring the wine over the fish right before baking.

....

Per serving: Calories: 267; Total fat: 10g; Total carbs: 4g; Fiber: 1g; Sugar: 5g; Protein: 33g; Sodium: 257mg

Beef and Broccoli with Oil-and-Garlic Sauce ▸ *page 91*

Chapter 6

🌿

POULTRY AND MEAT

CHICKEN NOODLE SOUP

**FREEZER-FRIENDLY,
MAKE-AHEAD, ONE-POT**

Serves 4

Prep time: 10 minutes

Cook time: 20 minutes

2 tablespoons extra-virgin
  olive oil

1 pound boneless, skinless
  chicken breasts, cut into
  bite-size pieces

½ teaspoon kosher salt

¼ teaspoon freshly ground
  black pepper

1 large onion,
  coarsely chopped

3 garlic cloves, crushed

5 cups chicken broth
  (page 116) or store-bought

3 cups water

1 pound frozen mixed
  vegetables

6 ounces small
  gluten-free pasta

Warm, hearty, and heavy on healthy ingredients, this chicken noodle soup is perfect for a cold day. Many studies have been done on the effects of chicken soup, with inconclusive results; nonetheless, I challenge anyone to say that chicken soup is not good for the soul. This version uses frozen veggies and premade chicken broth for a quicker soup that packs in lots of flavor. It can be made with any small pasta of your choice, such as quadretti, elbows, or small shells.

1. In a pot, heat the oil over medium-high heat.

2. Once the oil is hot, add the chicken, along with the salt and pepper. Sauté for 5 minutes.

3. Add the onion and garlic. Continue to cook for another 2 minutes or until fond (brown bits) starts to collect at the bottom and the chicken is browned.

4. Pour in the broth and water. Bring to a boil.

5. Add the vegetables and pasta. You may also want to add another pinch of salt and pepper.

6. Cook, uncovered, until the vegetables are tender and the pasta is cooked through, 8 to 10 minutes.

7.   Ladle into bowls and serve.

Tip: The use of frozen vegetables adds liquid to the soup, so do not add more broth or water than directed. If you would like to have a single serving and save the rest for later, remove the excess broth to a container and put it in refrigerator. Cook a small amount of noodles in the soup and serve immediately.

....

Per serving: Calories: 477; Total fat: 13g; Total carbs: 54g; Fiber: 7g; Sugar: 3g; Protein: 36g; Sodium: 599mg

GROUND TURKEY VEGETABLE SOUP

**FREEZER-FRIENDLY,
MAKE-AHEAD, ONE-POT**

Serves 4

Prep time: 5 minutes

Cook time: 20 minutes

2 tablespoons extra-virgin
olive oil

1 pound lean ground turkey

1 onion, finely chopped

2 garlic cloves, minced

6 cups chicken broth
(page 116) or store-bought

3 cups frozen mixed vegetables

1 (15-ounce) can cannellini
beans, drained and rinsed

Kosher salt

Freshly ground black pepper

1 cup coarsely chopped fresh
or frozen spinach

Warm, wholesome, and loaded with turkey, beans, and vegetables, this savory soup is a healthy meal that you can make with ingredients you already have at home. In addition to being quite comforting, this soup helps reduce pain-causing inflammation in the body.

1. In a pot, heat the oil over medium-high heat.

2. Add the turkey and use a wooden spoon to break into small pieces as it browns. Cook for 5 minutes or until no longer pink.

3. Toss in the onion and garlic. Cook while stirring for another 5 minutes.

4. Pour in the broth and bring to a boil.

5. Add the mixed vegetables, beans, and a generous pinch of salt and pepper. Let boil for 8 minutes.

6. Add the spinach and cook for another minute or until wilted.

7. Ladle the soup into bowls and serve.

Tip: Any leafy greens can be used in place of the spinach. Cannellini beans can be swapped with canned navy beans (also called great northern beans).

Per serving: Calories: 508; Total fat: 23g; Total carbs: 32g; Fiber: 9g; Sugar: 7g; Protein: 44g; Sodium: 439mg

GRILLED STEAK SALAD

MAKE-AHEAD

Serves 2
Prep time: 15 minutes
Cook time: 10 minutes

FOR THE SALAD

2 (6-ounce) flat iron steaks
(also called flat blade steak)
or steak of choice

1 teaspoon kosher salt

½ teaspoon freshly ground
black pepper

4 cups chopped butter lettuce

2 cups fresh or frozen spinach

½ cup pomegranate seeds

FOR THE VINAIGRETTE

2 tablespoons avocado oil

2 tablespoons apple
cider vinegar

1 tablespoon honey

Kosher salt

Freshly ground black pepper

This grilled steak salad is loaded with nutritious greens and pomegranate seeds, which add a fresh, fruity burst and vitamin C to every forkful. Vitamin C is a powerful antioxidant, which is particularly helpful during a flare-up. This is a great way to enjoy steak on occasion, among crisp greens lightly dressed with a vinaigrette that boasts a sweet earthiness accompanied by bright acidity.

TO MAKE THE SALAD

1. Season the steaks liberally with salt and pepper. Lay them on a paper towel to rest for 15 minutes, covering them with another paper towel on top to absorb any juices.

2. Heat a skillet over medium-high heat. Pat the steaks dry and sear for about 4 to 5 minutes per side, until the internal temperature reaches 140°F for medium rare.

3. While steak is sitting, combine the lettuce, spinach, and pomegranate seeds in a salad bowl and toss.

4. Slice or chop the steak, then add to the salad.

continued...

GRILLED STEAK SALAD *continued*

TO MAKE THE VINAIGRETTE

5. Whisk together the oil, vinegar, honey, salt, and pepper.

6. Drizzle dressing over the salad and toss.

Tip: If possible, purchase grass-fed beef. The steak can be made in advance, or you can even use leftovers from last night's barbecue. Lemon or lime juice can be substituted for the apple cider vinegar.

....

Per serving: Calories: 518; Total fat: 34g; Total carbs: 21g; Fiber: 4g; Sugar: 16g; Protein: 35g; Sodium: 1,340mg

TURKEY AND AVOCADO COLLARD GREEN WRAP

MAKE-AHEAD

Serves 2

Prep time: 10 minutes

Cook time: 12 minutes

1 tablespoon extra-virgin olive oil or avocado oil

1 pound turkey breast cutlets, cut into 1-inch chunks

½ teaspoon kosher salt

¼ teaspoon freshly ground black pepper

¼ teaspoon onion powder

⅛ teaspoon dried sage

1 garlic clove, minced

2 avocados, sliced

Juice of ½ lemon or 1 tablespoon bottled lemon juice

4 large collard green leaves, stemmed

These no-fuss wraps can be enjoyed at home or on-the-go. Raw collard leaves are nourishing, and their assertive and chewy texture adds more to a meal than a bland store-bought wrap. You can dip each leaf in boiling water for 20 seconds and then into an ice bath for a softer texture. The tender turkey seasoned with a bit of sage imparts a earthy aroma.

1. In a large skillet, heat the oil over medium heat.

2. Season the turkey with salt, pepper, onion powder, and sage.

3. Transfer to the skillet and cook for 7 minutes, stirring occasionally.

4. Toss in the garlic and continue to cook for 5 minutes. Cover the skillet for 3 more minutes, then remove from the heat.

5. Drizzle the avocados with lemon juice.

6. Divide the turkey evenly among the collard leaves and top with avocado. Wrap tightly and serve.

Tip: These wraps can be made up to 2 days in advance. Just wrap before refrigeration.

....

Per serving: Calories: 556; Total fat: 29g; Total carbs: 17g; Fiber: 12g; Sugar: 1g; Protein: 61g; Sodium: 723mg

TURMERIC CHICKEN WITH SPINACH AND BROWN RICE

FIVE INGREDIENTS OR LESS, FREEZER-FRIENDLY, MAKE-AHEAD

Serves 3
Prep time: 5 minutes
Cook time: 25 minutes

1 cup parboiled whole grain brown rice

6 ounces fresh baby spinach

¼ cup raisins

Salt

Freshly ground black pepper

1 pound boneless, skinless chicken breasts

1 tablespoon extra-virgin olive oil

1 teaspoon turmeric

The turmeric in this recipe shines through as the anti-inflammatory ingredient. The spinach and raisins complement the fragrant chicken beautifully to make this dish a complete meal that will delight your taste buds. Parboiled brown rice is a great way to get whole grains in without the lengthy cook time. For even less time, look in your grocery's freezer section for frozen brown rice, which just requires reheating.

1. Preheat the oven to 400°F.

2. Cook the brown rice according to the package directions. While still warm, remove it from the heat and mix in the spinach and raisins. Season with salt and pepper and set aside.

3. While the rice is cooking, coat the chicken breasts in oil, turmeric, salt, and pepper. Put chicken on a parchment-lined baking sheet and bake for 25 minutes, until cooked through.

4. To serve, spoon the rice and chicken onto plates.

Tip: This dish can be put into airtight containers in individual portions for meal prepping. Keep it in the refrigerator for up to 3 days or in the freezer for up to 3 months. For added flavor, season the chicken with garlic powder.

....

Per serving: Calories: 502; Total fat: 11g; Total carbs: 63g; Fiber: 4g; Sugar: 9g; Protein: 40g; Sodium: 119mg

SHREDDED CHICKEN TACOS

FREEZER-FRIENDLY, ONE-POT

Serves 3

Prep time: 7 minutes
Cook time: 20 minutes

1 tablespoon extra-virgin olive oil or avocado oil

1 pound boneless, skinless chicken breasts

1 teaspoon kosher salt

½ teaspoon freshly ground black pepper

¼ teaspoon ground cumin

¾ cup chicken broth (page 116) or vegetable broth (page 115)

½ cup shredded lettuce *(optional)*

½ cup diced avocado *(optional)*

¼ cup chopped red onion *(optional)*

¼ cup shredded vegan cheese *(optional)*

This shredded chicken taco recipe is simple from start to finish. The chicken simmers in broth that infuses it with flavor, adds moisture, and helps it fall apart easily. Just add your favorite taco toppings! I recommend nutritious lettuce, avocado for some good fat, and diced onion to help fight inflammation.

1. In a large saucepan, heat the oil over medium-high heat.

2. Season both sides of the chicken with salt, pepper, and cumin.

3. Put the chicken into the skillet and brown for 4 minutes per side.

4. Pour in the broth, reduce the heat to medium-low, and simmer, covered, for 12 minutes.

5. Remove the chicken from the pan and shred with two forks.

6. Fill the taco shells with the chicken.

7. Top with the lettuce, avocado, onion, and cheese (if using) and serve.

Tip: Leftover shredded chicken can be refrigerated for 4 days or frozen for up to 3 months. Additional garnishes could be corn salsa, shredded cabbage, or plant-based sour cream.

....

Per serving: Calories: 343; Total fat: 14g; Total carbs: 17g; Fiber: 2g; Sugar: 1g; Protein: 36g; Sodium: 975mg

CORIANDER-SPICED CHICKEN WITH CELERIAC

ONE-POT

Serves 2

Prep time: 5 minutes

Cook time: 25 minutes

8 to 10 baby carrots

2 medium celery roots (celeriac), peeled and cut into 1½-inch pieces

2 tablespoons extra-virgin olive oil

Kosher salt

Freshly ground black pepper

2 (6-ounce) boneless, skinless chicken breasts, thinly cut

2 garlic cloves, minced

½ teaspoon ground coriander

¼ teaspoon ground cumin

1 lemon, sliced

Chicken may be an excellent source of lean protein, but celeriac is the real star of this recipe. Celery root is high in fiber, vitamin K, potassium, and more. It adds a buttery, almost earthiness to the dish, making this dish both healthy and delicious.

1. Preheat the oven to 400°F.

2. Put the carrots and celery root onto a rimmed baking sheet. Drizzle with oil, season with salt and pepper, and toss.

3. Roast for 10 minutes.

4. Season both sides of the chicken with salt and pepper and add to the baking sheet.

5. Toss in the garlic, coriander, and cumin over the pan. Top with lemon slices.

6. Roast for 15 minutes or until the chicken is cooked through and the celeriac is tender and golden brown.

Tip: To peel celeriac, slice the root end off, place the flat end on the cutting board, and hold the stem with one hand as you cut from top to bottom, working your way around the bulb.

Per serving: Calories: 411; Total fat: 19g; Total carbs: 22g; Fiber: 5g; Sugar: 5g; Protein: 41g; Sodium: 265mg

BEEF LETTUCE CUPS

MAKE-AHEAD, ONE-POT

Serves 4
Prep time: 6 minutes
Cook time: 15 minutes

1 tablespoon extra-virgin olive
 oil or avocado oil

1 pound lean ground beef

1 yellow onion, chopped

2 garlic cloves, grated

½ teaspoon kosher salt

¼ teaspoon freshly ground
 black pepper

1 teaspoon soy sauce

16 butter lettuce leaves

Chopped fresh cilantro,
 for garnish

The secret to delicious lettuce cups is a well-seasoned filling. To achieve that, you need some fat, onion for sweetness, garlic for pungency, and a few other additions for depth. For this recipe, soy sauce is used to play up the flavor of the beef but can be swapped for tamari or coconut aminos for a soy-free version. Buying grass-fed beef will improve the nutrition profile of this dish.

1. In a skillet, heat the oil over medium-high heat.

2. Add the ground beef and use a wooden spoon to break the meat into small pieces as it browns, about 8 minutes.

3. Add the onion, garlic, salt, and pepper. Continue to cook, stirring, for another 3 minutes.

4. Stir in the soy sauce and reduce the heat to medium-low. Let cook for another 3 minutes.

5. Remove from the heat, spoon the beef into lettuce cups, and garnish with cilantro.

Tip: The filling can be made up to 3 days in advance. Just spoon into the lettuce cups and garnish with cilantro before serving.

....

Per serving: Calories: 292; Total fat: 16g; Total carbs: 4g; Fiber: 1g; Sugar: 1g; Protein: 31g; Sodium: 438mg

CHICKEN WITH ZUCCHINI NOODLES AND CAULIFLOWER "ALFREDO"

FREEZER-FRIENDLY, MAKE-AHEAD

Serves 4
Prep Time: 5 minutes
Cook Time: 27 minutes

FOR THE "ALFREDO" SAUCE

½ head cauliflower, coarsely chopped

1 teaspoon avocado oil

1 yellow onion, chopped

2 garlic cloves, minced

¼ cup nutritional yeast

½ cup canned full-fat coconut milk

Juice of 1 lemon or 2 tablespoons bottled lemon juice

½ teaspoon salt

FOR THE CHICKEN AND ZUCCHINI NOODLES

1¼ pounds boneless, skinless chicken breast

1 tablespoon chopped fresh rosemary

¼ teaspoon garlic powder

¼ teaspoon salt

1 teaspoon avocado oil

1 (10-ounce) package fresh zucchini noodles or 2 medium zucchini, spiralized

Sometimes a little goes a long way, and that is certainly true when it comes to using fresh rosemary. This pungent herb appeals to the senses and can be an invigorating, true pick-me-up. This dish can be made ahead of time and assembled just before eating. The sauce is warm and tangy, offering a great compliment to the rosemary-infused chicken.

TO MAKE THE "ALFREDO" SAUCE

1. Put water in a pot fitted with a steaming basket. Fill to just below the basket and add the cauliflower to the basket. Steam the cauliflower until soft, about 10 minutes. Remove the basket and cauliflower and set aside. Discard the water.

2. Carefully wipe out the pot and return to the stove over medium-high heat. Pour in the oil, add the onion, and cook for 5 minutes, until translucent.

3. Lower the heat and add the garlic, cooking for another minute.

4. Put the cauliflower, onion, and garlic in a blender and add the yeast, coconut milk, lemon juice, and salt. Blend until smooth.

TO MAKE THE CHICKEN AND ZUCCHINI NOODLES

5. Season the chicken with the rosemary, garlic powder, and salt.

6. In a skillet, heat the oil over medium heat.

....

7. Add the chicken breasts to the pan and sauté for
    6 minutes per side, or until fully cooked through.
    Remove and slice the breasts.

8. Plate the zucchini noodles, topping with sliced
    chicken and cauliflower "Alfredo" sauce.

Tip: You can make this dish vegan by swapping tofu in for the
chicken. If you prefer your zucchini noodles cooked, you can
sauté them for 3 to 5 minutes after cooking the chicken. The
sauce can be made ahead and refrigerated in an airtight container
for up to 3 days, or frozen for up to 3 months.

....

Per serving: Calories: 313; Total fat: 12g; Total carbs: 15g; Fiber: 5g;
Sugar: 6g; Protein: 39g; Sodium: 539mg

ROTISSERIE CHICKEN WITH ASPARAGUS

FIVE INGREDIENTS OR LESS, FREEZER-FRIENDLY, MAKE-AHEAD

Serves 4
Prep time: 5 minutes
Cook time: 15 minutes

1 pound fresh or frozen asparagus, ends trimmed (about 3 cups)

3 tablespoons extra-virgin olive oil, divided

½ teaspoon salt, divided

1 pound whole cooked rotisserie chicken, skin and bones removed

12 ounces frozen cauliflower rice

This recipe takes a precooked supermarket chicken and turns it into a well-rounded, tasty meal with minimal effort. Frozen cauliflower rice is easier on the jaw because it is already chopped into fine pieces, which eliminates some "chew" work. Asparagus contains the flavonoids quercetin, isorhamnetin, and kaempferol, which have anti-inflammatory properties.

1. Preheat the oven to 400°F. Line a baking sheet with parchment paper.

2. Place the asparagus on the baking sheet in a single layer. Drizzle 1½ tablespoons of oil and ¼ teaspoon of salt on top, and toss to coat. Roast in the oven until slightly crisp, about 15 minutes.

3. In the meantime, put the chicken in an oven-safe baking dish and cover. Bake in the oven for 10 minutes. Set aside.

4. While the asparagus and the chicken are in the oven, put the cauliflower rice in a microwave-safe bowl. Microwave on high for 2 minutes, stir, then microwave about 2 minutes more, or until fully heated.

5. Add the remaining 1½ tablespoons of oil and ¼ teaspoon of salt to the cauliflower rice and mix.

6. Divide the asparagus, cauliflower rice, and chicken onto plates.

Tip: Use this recipe for batch cooking by dividing leftovers into containers and freezing. You can substitute broccoli florets or sliced zucchini rounds for the asparagus. Some supermarkets might add salt to the seasoning on the chicken skin, which is why removing the skin is recommended.

Per serving: Calories: 346; Total fat: 22g; Total carbs: 8g; Fiber: 4g; Sugar: 4g; Protein: 33g; Sodium: 709mg

LEMON-OREGANO CHICKEN

FIVE INGREDIENTS OR LESS

Serves 4

Prep time: 5 minutes

Cook time: 20 minutes

4 (6-ounce) boneless, skinless chicken breasts, pounded to even thickness

2 tablespoons extra-virgin olive oil

Juice of 1 lemon or 2 tablespoons bottled lemon juice

1 teaspoon kosher salt

1 tablespoon fresh oregano

The contrast of tart lemon and peppery oregano has a special way of enhancing plain chicken breasts. Although lean and packed with protein, white meat is a blank slate. For this recipe, all you need is chicken, olive oil for fat and depth of flavor, fresh oregano, lemon, and salt to make a flavorful main to serve with your favorite side.

1. Preheat the oven to 400°F.

2. Put the chicken into an ungreased baking dish.

3. In a bowl, whisk together the oil, lemon juice, and salt, then add the oregano.

4. Pour the mixture over the chicken and bake for 10 minutes.

5. Baste the chicken with the pan juices and bake for another 10 minutes or until the chicken breasts are opaque and no pink remains.

6. Serve with your favorite side dish.

Tip: Fresh oregano can be replaced with 1 teaspoon of dried oregano. Broil for 3 minutes to develop more color on the top of each chicken breast. Add freshly ground black pepper to play up oregano's peppery bite.

Per serving: Calories: 260; Total fat: 11g; Total carbs: 1g; Fiber: 1g; Sugar: <1g; Protein: 38g; Sodium: 666mg

BEEF AND BROCCOLI WITH OIL-AND-GARLIC SAUCE

....

FIVE INGREDIENTS OR LESS, MAKE-AHEAD, ONE-POT

Serves 4
Prep time: 7 minutes
Cook time: 16 minutes

FOR THE BEEF AND BROCCOLI

1 tablespoon avocado oil

16 ounces flank steak, cut into thin slices against the grain

Kosher salt

Freshly ground black pepper

32 ounces fresh broccoli florets (about 4 cups)

FOR THE SAUCE

¼ cup extra-virgin olive oil

1 tablespoon finely chopped garlic

2 tablespoons chopped fresh flat-leaf parsley

½ teaspoon kosher salt

The sauce in this dish is fragrant, as the garlic infuses its flavor into the oil. The addition of fresh parsley offers a crisp taste, and the quick sear of the thinly sliced beef allows it to absorb the garlic sauce, creating a complete meal quickly and easily.

TO MAKE THE BEEF AND BROCCOLI

1. In a large skillet, heat the oil over medium-high heat.

2. Add the flank steak slices, cooking 3 to 4 minutes on each side. Season with salt and pepper.

3. Add in the broccoli, reduce the heat to medium, and cook for 5 minutes.

TO MAKE THE SAUCE

4. Add the oil, garlic, and parsley to the pan with the steak and broccoli and cook over medium heat for another 2 minutes.

5. Divide into bowls and serve.

Tip: For a more pronounced flavor, use a garlic press to mash the garlic. Be careful not to burn the garlic when sautéing. This dish can be refrigerated for up to 3 days.

....

Per serving: Calories: 353; Total fat: 25g; Total carbs: 5g; Fiber: 2g; Sugar: 1g; Protein: 20g; Sodium: 378mg

BEEF AND EGG BOWL

**FIVE INGREDIENTS OR
LESS, MAKE-AHEAD,
ONE-POT**

Serves 4
Prep time: 5 minutes
Cook time: 15 minutes

1 tablespoon olive oil

½ pound extra-lean
ground beef

1½ cups chopped fresh
kale leaves

2 eggs

1 avocado, cubed

2 tablespoons
nutritional yeast

This delightful combination of eggs and beef with nutritious kale allows you to enjoy the red meat flavor while also getting a serving of omega-3-rich greens, helping to decrease inflammation. Having red meat as a mixture, rather than the star of the meal, helps you get used to eating less of it. It is okay to enjoy red meat on occasion, and this bowl is a great way to do so. Of course, a vegan "beef" can be substituted for the ground beef.

1. In a skillet, heat the oil over medium heat.

2. Add the beef, breaking it up as you sauté. Cook for about 10 minutes, or until the beef is cooked through.

3. Drain any fat from the pan by tilting the pan and using a spoon to collect it.

4. Add the kale to the pan with the beef. Crack the eggs over the mixture and stir to combine. Cook for 5 minutes, or until the kale is wilted and the eggs are cooked.

5. Divide the mixture among bowls and top with the avocado and yeast to serve.

Tip: Buying grass-fed beef will improve the nutrition content of the meat. This recipe can be made in advance and reheated and assembled later. The avocado should be cut right before serving.

Per serving: Calories: 209; Total fat: 14g; Total carbs: 5g; Fiber: 4g; Sugar: <1g; Protein: 18g; Sodium: 66mg

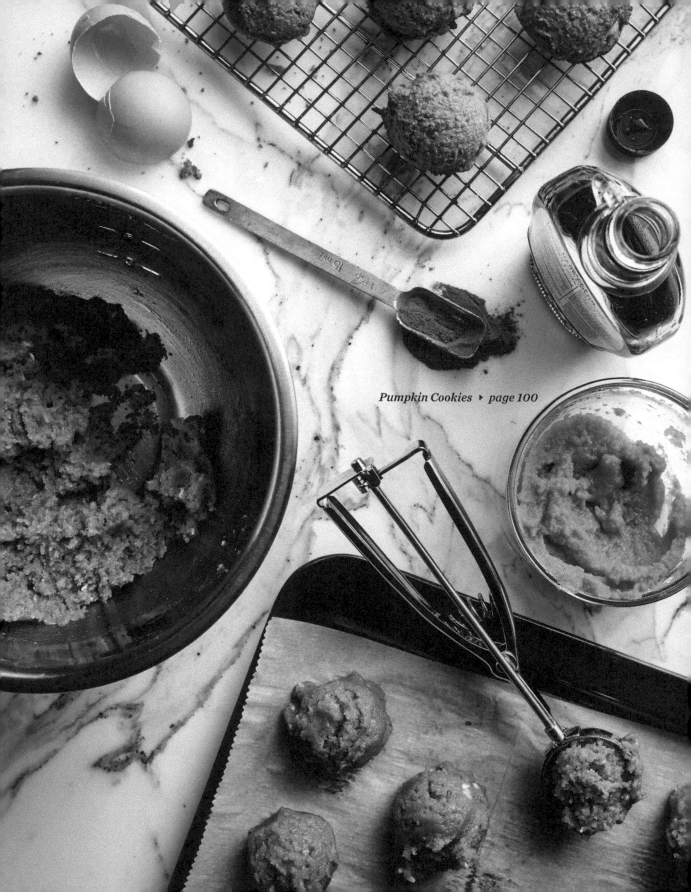

Pumpkin Cookies ▸ *page 100*

Chapter 7

🌿

SNACKS AND DESSERTS

CHOCOLATE-COVERED WALNUTS

FIVE INGREDIENTS OR LESS, FREEZER-FRIENDLY, MAKE-AHEAD, VEGAN

Serves 5

Prep time: 5 to 10 minutes

6 ounces dark chocolate, 70-percent cocoa or higher

1 cup walnut halves

Kosher salt

Cinnamon for sprinkling

Walnuts are a great source of anti-inflammatory omega-3 fatty acids. They are also low in FODMAPs, a group of small-chain carbohydrates that fibro warriors may want to avoid. Topped with salt for flavor and cinnamon to add another anti-inflammatory layer, this special treat can be enjoyed as a snack or a dessert.

1. Line a baking sheet with parchment paper and set aside.

2. Put the chocolate in a glass bowl. Microwave on high for 1 minute. Stir with a rubber spatula. Microwave for 20-second intervals after the initial minute, stirring in between, until fully melted.

3. Add the walnut halves to the chocolate and stir gently until each walnut is fully coated.

4. Using a fork, pick up each walnut and place it on the lined baking sheet. Sprinkle the walnuts with the salt and cinnamon.

5. Put the tray in the refrigerator to cool until the chocolate has hardened, about 10 minutes. Remove the walnuts and store in an airtight container.

Tip: You can store your chocolate nuts in an airtight container in the refrigerator for 4 weeks or freeze for 6 months. Substitute walnuts with pecans, if desired.

Per serving: Calories: 334; Total fat: 28g; Total carbs: 18g; Fiber: 5g; Sugar: 9g; Protein: 6g; Sodium: 7mg

CHOCOLATE, COCONUT, AND ALMOND COOKIE DOUGH BALLS

FREEZER-FRIENDLY, MAKE AHEAD, VEGAN

Makes 16 dough balls
Prep time: 12 minutes

1 cup almond flour

1 cup unsweetened dried coconut flakes

1 cup creamy almond butter, no salt or sugar added

⅓ cup hemp seeds

2 tablespoons unsweetened cacao powder

2 tablespoons water

1 tablespoon maple syrup

1½ teaspoons vanilla extract

Rich and chocolatey with nutty notes, these cookie dough balls have it all. The chewy treats offer the same satisfaction as scooping into a log of cookie dough, minus the guilt! With each bite you get the satisfyingly intense flavor of real chocolate. The almonds and coconut combined with the hemp seeds add texture variation, and the maple syrup brings just enough sweetness. Best of all, they taste even better the second day.

1. In a medium bowl, combine the flour, coconut, almond butter, hemp seeds, cacao powder, water, maple syrup, and vanilla. Mix with a rubber spatula until smooth.

2. Roll into 16 (1-inch) balls and place on a sheet pan. Chill in the freezer for 30 minutes.

3. Remove and store in an airtight container. Keep refrigerated or frozen until ready to eat.

Tip: If the mixture is a bit too sticky to handle, add another teaspoon of almond flour. Cookie dough balls can be stored in the refrigerator for up to 1 week. You can also freeze them for 6 months.

....

Per serving (1 ball): Calories: 194; Total fat: 17g; Total carbs: 7g; Fiber: 4g; Sugar: 2g; Protein: 6g; Sodium: 4mg

FROZEN BLUEBERRY YOGURT POPPERS

FIVE INGREDIENTS OR LESS, FREEZER-FRIENDLY, MAKE-AHEAD, VEGAN

Serves 4

Prep time: 30 minutes

2 cups blueberries, fresh
  or frozen

¼ cup plain dairy-free yogurt

This is an easy, nutrient-dense frozen dessert that is great for satisfying an ice cream craving. Keep it in the fridge, and when you hear the ice cream truck coming down your block, go ahead and reach for it! Blueberries contain polyphenols, which are known for their anti-inflammatory effect. This is particularly true of inflammation in the brain, according to one study published in 2014 in Neural Regeneration Research.

1. Line a baking sheet with parchment paper and set aside.

2. In a bowl, combine the blueberries and yogurt until the blueberries are well-coated.

3. Lifting them with a fork, transfer the individual yogurt-covered blueberries to the prepared baking sheet in an even layer.

4. Freeze for 30 minutes, then transfer to a freezer bag or a freezer-safe storage container. Store in the freezer until ready to eat.

Tip: These treats will defrost quickly, so take out only a few at a time. You can substitute blueberries with strawberry halves for a different flavor.

Per serving: Calories: 49; Total fat: 1g; Total carbs: 11g; Fiber: 2g; Sugar: 7g; Protein: 1g; Sodium: 4mg

AVOCADO-MINT SORBET

FIVE INGREDIENTS OR LESS, FREEZER-FRIENDLY, MAKE-AHEAD, ONE-POT, VEGETARIAN

Serves 4
Prep time: 5 minutes

1 cup diced frozen avocado

⅔ cup frozen pineapple

8 fresh mint leaves

1 tablespoon honey

Juice of 2 limes or ¼ cup bottled lime juice

Fresh mint paired with creamy avocado makes the ultimate sorbet. The lingering cooling effect of the fragrant herb is present in every spoonful, the avocado helps maintain its smooth yet icy texture, and frozen pineapple provides the sweet acidity you expect in a quality sorbet. Frozen fruit, mint leaves, a little natural sweetener, and a food processor are all you need to make a refreshing, ice-cold treat in minutes.

1. In a food processor or blender, combine the avocado, pineapple, mint, honey, and lime juice. Process until smooth.

2. Serve immediately or transfer to a freezer-safe container and chill in the freezer. Thaw slightly before serving.

Tip: Any frozen fruit can be used in place of the pineapple. If vegan, use maple syrup in place of honey. You can also use a small food processor or personal blender to make the sorbet.

Per serving: Calories: 92; Total fat: 5g; Total carbs: 14g; Fiber: 3g; Sugar: 6g; Protein: 1g; Sodium: 2mg

PUMPKIN COOKIES

**FREEZER-FRIENDLY,
MAKE-AHEAD,
VEGETARIAN**

Makes **12 cookies**
Prep time: **10 minutes**
Cook time: **20 minutes**

2 cups plus 2 tablespoons
  almond flour

⅓ cup 100-percent pure
  pumpkin puree

¼ cup almond butter, no salt
  or sugar added

2 tablespoons coconut oil

1 large egg

1 heaping tablespoon
  maple syrup

2 teaspoons vanilla extract

½ teaspoon baking powder

1 teaspoon ground cinnamon

¼ teaspoon ground nutmeg

⅛ teaspoon salt

The earthy, sweet taste of pumpkin and the warmth of the bold spices come through nicely in these soft and cakey cookies. Better yet, they are so easy to whip up! In addition to the nutritious pumpkin, the cookies are loaded with almonds via almond flour and butter, meaning more protein and healthy fat for you.

1. Preheat the oven to 350°F and line a baking sheet with parchment paper.

2. In a medium bowl, combine the almond flour, pumpkin, almond butter, oil, egg, maple syrup, vanilla, baking powder, cinnamon, nutmeg, and salt. Mix until a thick dough forms. Add more almond flour if the dough is too runny.

3. Scoop the dough in 2-tablespoon portions and place on a rimmed baking sheet.

4. Bake for 20 minutes or until golden brown.

5. Remove from the oven and let fully cool before serving.

Tip: For a vegan option, substitute the egg with the Flaxseed Egg Substitute (page 114). Cookies can be refrigerated for up to 1 week or put in an airtight container and stored in the freezer for up to 1 month.

Per serving (1 cookie): Calories: 184; Total fat: 16g; Total carbs: 7g; Fiber: 3g; Sugar: 3g; Protein: 6g; Sodium: 53mg

LIME AND OLIVE OIL MINI-CAKE

VEGETARIAN

Serves 1
Prep time: 5 minutes
Cook time: 20 minutes

1½ teaspoons extra-virgin olive oil, divided

3 tablespoons almond flour

2 tablespoons creamy sunflower butter, no sugar added

1 teaspoon flaxseed meal

½ tablespoon honey, plus more for garnish

1 teaspoon freshly squeezed or bottled lime juice

¼ teaspoon vanilla extract

Olive oil makes an exceptionally good cake because of the moisture it has to offer. Combine that with its great taste the result is phenomenal. Olive oil serves as a mild flavor base for this personal mini-cake, while the lime brightens it up with its fresh flavor. Additionally, honey is used for sweetness and adds another dimension of flavor to the cake, while also promoting browning.

1. Preheat the oven to 350°F and lightly grease a ramekin with ½ teaspoon of oil.

2. In a small bowl, mix the remaining 1 teaspoon of oil with the flour, sunflower butter, flaxseed, honey, lime juice, and vanilla.

3. Pour into the ramekin and spread in an even layer.

4. Put on a baking sheet and bake for 20 minutes.

5. Remove from the oven, lightly drizzle with more honey (if desired), and serve.

Tip: For best results, select a fruity olive oil. Fresh lime juice will give more flavor than juice from the bottle. A wide-glass jam jar, oven-safe mug, or greased muffin tin can be used in place of a ramekin.

....

Per serving (1 brownie): Calories: 426; Total fat: 36g; Total carbs: 21g; Fiber: 5g; Sugar: 13g; Protein: 11g; Sodium: 5mg

MAPLE-BANANA CHIA PUDDING

**FIVE INGREDIENTS OR
LESS, MAKE-AHEAD,
VEGAN**

Serves 2
Prep time: 5 minutes

1 ripe banana, mashed

1 cup unsweetened
  almond milk

2 tablespoons chia seeds

½ tablespoon maple syrup

1 teaspoon vanilla extract

*Maple-banana chia pudding is a make-ahead dessert
worth boasting about. Maple syrup and ripe banana
are joined by a hint of vanilla to create a thick, rich
pudding that's good for you. It is high in fiber, protein, omega-3s, and antioxidants, which everyone
needs in their diet. The banana flavor is at the fore-
front, the sweetness level is just right, and the chewy
bite of the chia seeds make it all the better.*

1. In a bowl, combine the banana, almond milk, chia
   seeds, maple syrup, and vanilla and stir.

2. Transfer to individual serving glasses.

3. Cover with plastic and chill in the refrigerator for
   6 hours or overnight. The pudding will thicken as
   it chills.

Tip: The colder the pudding gets, the better it tastes! Pudding can
be made up to 2 days in advance.

Per serving: Calories: 150; Total fat: 5g; Total carbs: 23g; Fiber: 7g;
Sugar: 11g; Protein: 3g; Sodium: 87mg

STRAWBERRIES WITH MACADAMIA NUT DIP

FIVE INGREDIENTS OR LESS, MAKE-AHEAD, ONE-POT, VEGAN

Serves 4

Prep time: 3 minutes

1 cup macadamia nuts, presoaked at least 30 minutes

1⅓ tablespoons coconut oil, melted

1½ cups whole strawberries

Macadamia nuts are high in fat, but it is mostly monounsaturated, which is considered heart-healthy. Make this quick-and-easy nut dip to get your daily serving of manganese, which can help regulate blood sugar and reduce inflammation. The pairing of the sweet tartness of strawberries with the richness of macadamia nuts is pure heaven.

1. In a food processor or blender, combine the macadamia nuts and oil. Process until smooth and creamy. If needed, add water until the desired consistency is reached. It should be thick like a dip.

2. Transfer to a bowl. Serve with the strawberries.

Tip: The dip can be refrigerated for up to 2 weeks. For a nut-free version, use sunflower seed butter instead of macadamia nuts.

....

Per serving: Calories: 299; Total fat: 30g; Total carbs: 9g; Fiber: 4g; Sugar: 4g; Protein: 3g; Sodium: 2mg

CHERRY-BALSAMIC GLAZED YOGURT

**FIVE INGREDIENTS OR
LESS, VEGAN**

Serves 4
Prep time: 2 minutes
Cook time: 15 minutes

2 cups frozen cherries

¼ cup maple syrup

½ cup balsamic vinegar

3 cups unsweetened
    coconut yogurt

¼ cup hemp seeds

This recipe will satisfy your sweet tooth without filling you with sugar. Sweet and tangy notes from the combination of cherries and balsamic vinegar are a delight to the palate. While vinegar in a dessert might seem out of place, it is commonly used by many a fancy chef. You can serve this to guests and wow them with your culinary expertise!

1. In a small saucepan, cook the cherries, maple syrup, and vinegar over medium heat. Simmer for 10 to 12 minutes, until the liquid has reduced by almost half, then remove from the heat and cool.

2. Divide the yogurt into bowls or containers. Top with the glaze and hemp seeds and serve.

Tip: Be sure to allow the glaze to reduce by half; this will soften the flavor of the vinegar. To make this sugar-free, substitute the maple syrup with Lakanto maple-flavored syrup.

Per serving: Calories: 258; Total fat: 10g; Total carbs: 39g; Fiber: 4g; Sugar: 26g; Protein: 5g; Sodium: 44mg

AVOCADO BROWNIES

MAKE-AHEAD, VEGAN

*Makes **8 brownies***
*Prep time: **10 minutes***
*Cook time: **20 minutes***

1 large avocado, mashed

2 large eggs

½ cup nut butter, no salt or
   sugar added

1 heaping tablespoon
   maple syrup

1 teaspoon vanilla extract

½ cup almond flour

½ cup unsweetened
   cacao powder

½ teaspoon baking soda

Pinch salt

¼ cup cacao nibs

*These avocado brownies are actually good for you!
The avocado makes these brownies decadent, cacao
powder and nibs deliver the chocolate you crave
(minus the sugar), and your favorite nut butter adds
healthy fat.*

1. Preheat the oven to 350°F and line a 9-inch square
    baking pan with parchment paper.

2. In the bowl of a food processor, combine the
    avocado, eggs, nut butter, maple syrup, and vanilla.
    Process until smooth.

3. In a mixing bowl, combine the almond flour, cacao
    powder, baking soda, and salt. Add the wet ingre-
    dients and stir until well combined. Fold in the
    cacao nibs.

4. Pour the batter into the prepared pan and smooth
    in an even layer.

5. Bake for 20 minutes or until a toothpick comes out
    clean when inserted in the center.

6. Let cool for 30 minutes to an hour, then cut into
    8 squares.

Tip: You can also mash the avocado, then whisk it into the wet
ingredients. This will have no effect on taste, but the batter will
be lumpier.

· · · · · · · · · · · · · · · ·

Per serving (1 brownie): Calories: 249; Total fat: 21g; Total carbs: 12g;
Fiber: 8g; Sugar: 3g; Protein: 8g; Sodium: 98mg

WARM APPLES WITH ALMOND BUTTER

FIVE INGREDIENTS OR LESS, MAKE-AHEAD, ONE-POT, VEGAN

Serves 2
Prep time: 3 minutes
Cook time: 10 minutes

2 teaspoons coconut oil

2 apples, Granny Smith or Honeycrisp, diced

1 teaspoon cinnamon

¼ cup almond butter

Sometimes simplicity does the trick. In this easy-to-construct snack, the crisp apple flavor combined with the warm almond butter is comforting and filling. Try to use Ceylon cinnamon if you can find it. It is a better-quality cinnamon compared to the more common cassia cinnamon, with a milder flavor as well.

1. In a skillet, heat the oil over low heat.

2. Add the apples and sauté for 8 to 10 minutes, until softened. Sprinkle with cinnamon and remove from the heat.

3. To serve, divide apples into bowls and top with almond butter.

Tip: Substitute any nut- or seed-based butter of your choice. Leave the skin on the apples for extra fiber.

Per serving (1 cup): Calories: 330; Total fat: 22g; Total carbs: 32g; Fiber: 8g; Sugar: 20g; Protein: 7g; Sodium: 73mg

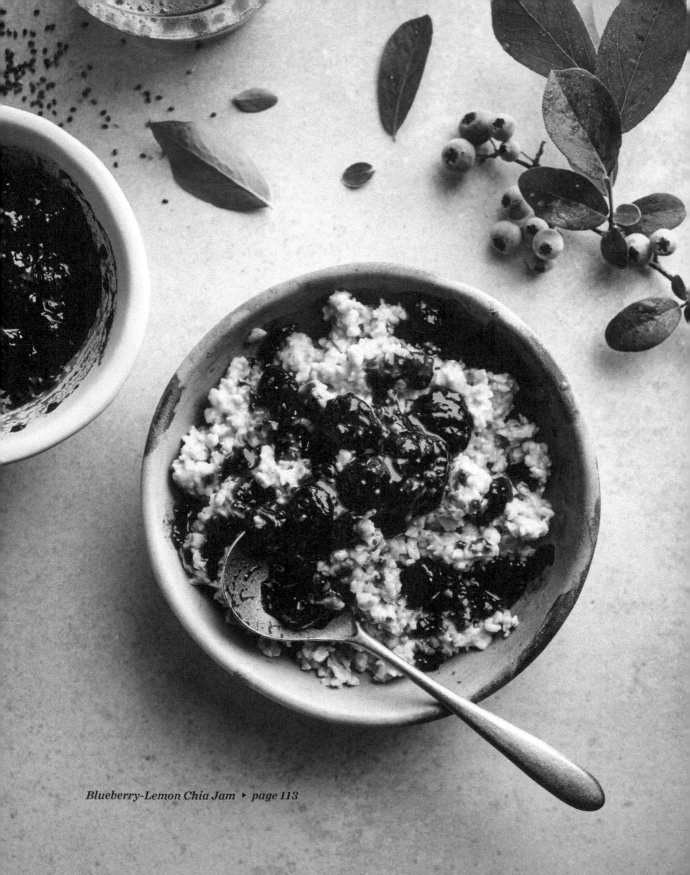

Blueberry-Lemon Chia Jam ▸ *page 113*

Chapter 8

🌿

BASICS

TAHINA SAUCE

FIVE INGREDIENTS OR LESS, FREEZER-FRIENDLY, MAKE-AHEAD, ONE-POT, VEGAN

Serves 12
Prep time: 2 minutes

3 large garlic cloves

Juice of 3 lemons or ⅓ cup bottled lemon juice

2 teaspoons kosher salt

2 cups tahini paste

1 teaspoon ground cumin

1 cup water, plus more for thinning

Tahina is a Middle Eastern condiment that goes with anything. Drizzle over chickpeas, roasted vegetables, tofu, or meat—you can't go wrong! This is a favorite in my house; I make it every week. The lemony creaminess of this sauce is absolute heaven, and its health factor is boosted by sesame's excellent anti-inflammatory properties.

1. In a blender, combine the garlic, lemon juice, salt, tahini paste, cumin, and 1 cup of water. Puree until smooth, about 1 minute.

2. Taste and adjust the seasonings as needed. If the mixture is too thick, add more water, 2 tablespoons at a time. For a thicker sauce, add less water. For dressing, thin out more. The mixture will thicken when refrigerated.

Tip: Tahini paste can be found in the Middle Eastern section of your grocery store. It might settle in the container with the oil on the top; just mix before measuring it out. This sauce will keep in the refrigerator for 1 week. Freeze for longer storage.

Per serving: Calories: 242; Total fat: 22g; Total carbs: 10g; Fiber: 4g; Sugar: 1g; Protein: 7g; Sodium: 440mg

DAIRY-FREE TZATZIKI

MAKE-AHEAD, ONE-POT, VEGAN

Serves 4

Prep time: 2 minutes

1 cup coconut or soy yogurt

1 tablespoon extra-virgin olive oil

1 English cucumber, seeded, finely grated, and drained

1 garlic clove, minced

2 tablespoons chopped fresh dill

1 teaspoon chopped fresh mint

Juice of ½ lemon or 1 tablespoon bottled lemon juice

½ teaspoon kosher salt

½ teaspoon freshly ground black pepper

A traditionally Greek condiment, this tzatziki recipe is cool and refreshing. The fresh herbs are rich in antioxidants, and the plant-based yogurt has plenty of good bacteria to help keep your gut healthy. Recent research shows that our brain health actually begins in the stomach, so giving your gut everything it needs to maintain its microbiota is a wise choice. Spoon some tzatziki onto your veggies, meat, or beans to elevate even the simplest of dishes.

In a bowl, whisk together the yogurt, oil, cucumber, garlic, dill, mint, lemon juice, salt, and pepper. Cover with plastic and chill.

Tip: Tzatziki is best when chilled for at least an hour, so consider making it in advance. To drain the cucumber, put it into a fine-mesh strainer placed over a bowl and let drain for 1 hour.

Per serving: Calories: 67; Total fat: 5g; Total carbs: 5g; Fiber: 2g; Sugar: 1g; Protein: 1g; Sodium: 307mg

ALMOND "FETA CHEESE" WHEEL

**FIVE INGREDIENTS OR
LESS, MAKE-AHEAD,
VEGAN**

Serves 8
Prep time: 7 minutes
Cook time: 20 minutes

1½ cups almond flour
(without skins)

¼ cup fresh or bottled
lemon juice

3 tablespoons extra-virgin
olive oil

1 garlic clove

1 teaspoon salt

*Dairy cheese is thought to cause inflammation and
pain, so having a vegan option is helpful. There
are many vegan cheeses you can purchase, but this
homemade version is easy and delicious. Made from
almond flour, this recipe is high in magnesium, an
essential mineral for nerve, bone, and muscle health.
I dare you to find a more delicious feta alternative!*

1. Preheat the oven to 350°F. Line a baking sheet with
   parchment paper and set aside.

2. In a blender or food processor, combine the
   almond flour, lemon juice, oil, garlic, and salt. Puree
   until smooth.

3. Remove the mixture from the blender and shape
   it into a ball. Place the ball on the prepared baking
   sheet and flatten the top.

4. Bake in the oven for 20 minutes. Let cool, then slice
   or crumble to serve.

Tip: For added flavor, include fresh chopped herbs in your cheese
mixture. This "cheese" wheel will keep in the fridge for 10 days in
an airtight container. It is best enjoyed on crackers or sprinkled
on top of a salad.

Per serving: Calories: 167; Total fat: 16g; Total carbs: 5g; Fiber: 2g;
Sugar: 1g; Protein: 5g; Sodium: 303mg

BLUEBERRY-LEMON CHIA JAM

**FIVE INGREDIENTS OR
LESS, FREEZER-FRIENDLY,
MAKE AHEAD, ONE-POT,
VEGAN**

Serves 8
*Prep time: **2 minutes***
*Cook time: **20 minutes***

1 cup frozen blueberries

**Juice of 1 lemon or
2 tablespoons bottled
lemon juice**

1 tablespoon maple syrup

2 teaspoons chia seeds

*This delicious jam is so much healthier than any
kind you can buy, and the best part is that it is loaded
with real fruit. Chia seeds offer omega-3 fatty acids,
fiber, protein, and antioxidants. Spread this jam on
crackers or toast, or swirl it in your oatmeal.*

1. In a saucepan, heat the blueberries, lemon juice,
   and maple syrup on medium-low heat. When the
   mixture starts to bubble, reduce the heat to low
   and simmer for 15 minutes.

2. Add the chia seeds and cook for 5 more minutes.
   The mixture will start to thicken.

3. Remove from the heat and let cool. Transfer to a
   glass jar with a lid.

Tip: This jam can be kept in the refrigerator for 7 days or frozen
for longer storage. For a sugar-free alternative, substitute
Lakanto maple-flavored syrup for the maple syrup.

Per serving: Calories: 27; Total fat: 1g; Total carbs: 6g; Fiber: 1g;
Sugar: 4g; Protein: <1g; Sodium: 1mg

FLAXSEED EGG SUBSTITUTE

FIVE INGREDIENTS OR LESS, MAKE-AHEAD, ONE-POT, VEGAN

Serves 1

Prep time: 6 minutes

2½ tablespoons water

1 tablespoon ground
   flaxseed meal

For those who want to try a vegan approach, it is useful to know how to substitute flaxseed for eggs in any recipe. One study published in 2000 in the Scandinavian Journal of Rheumatology *compared patients who were on a three-month vegan diet with patients eating an omnivorous diet. Those on the vegan diet had a statistically significant reduction in their pain scale. While more research is needed, trying to eliminate animal sources of protein can be worth trying. This recipe below is for 1 egg. You can scale up depending on how many eggs you need.*

In a small bowl, combine the water and flaxseed meal. Stir and let rest for 5 minutes, until the mixture thickens.

Tip: This egg substitute will work well in baked goods such as pancakes, brownies, cookies, and muffins. For a recipe which requires firming, such as a pumpkin pie, store-bought egg substitutes might work best.

....

Per serving: Calories: 40; Total fat: 3g; Total carbs: 2g; Fiber: 2g; Sugar: 0g; Protein: 2g; Sodium: 0mg

QUICK AND EASY VEGETABLE BROTH

MAKE-AHEAD, ONE-POT, VEGAN

Makes 8 cups
Prep time: 5 minutes
Cook time: 25 minutes

9 cups water

1 onion, quartered

2 celery stalks, quartered

2 carrots, quartered

3 garlic cloves, peeled and halved lengthwise

¼ cup dried mushrooms

2 bay leaves

1 tablespoon peppercorns

2 thyme sprigs or 1 teaspoon dried thyme

This recipe can be made in a pinch when you need some broth for another recipe, or if you aren't feeling your best and want a warm, aromatic soup to heat you up. Bay leaves and peppercorns add depth of flavor, and dried mushrooms lend a smoky element to this satisfying broth. Dried mushrooms are also an excellent source of B vitamins, which are necessary for energy production.

1. In a pot, combine the water, onion, celery, carrot, garlic, mushrooms, bay leaves, peppercorns, and thyme and bring to a boil over high heat. Reduce the heat to low and simmer, uncovered, for 25 minutes. The mixture should bubble slightly while simmering.

2. To use the broth, discard all the solids with a hand-held mesh strainer or tongs. Remember to get the peppercorns out, too!

Tip: You can add any leftover veggies you have to this mixture, either fresh or frozen. For extra flavor, you can add 1 tablespoon of miso paste at the end.

....

Per serving (1 cup): Calories: 14; Total fat: <1g; Total carbs: 3g; Fiber: 1g; Sugar: 1g; Protein: <1g; Sodium: 10mg

CHICKEN BROTH

FREEZER-FRIENDLY, MAKE-AHEAD

*Makes **10 cups***
*Prep time: **5 minutes***
*Cook time: **1 hour and 35 minutes***

3 bone-in, skin-on chicken breast halves

1 large onion, quartered

5 garlic cloves, peeled

2 celery stalks

½ cup fresh flat-leaf parsley

¼ teaspoon salt

½ tablespoon freshly ground black pepper

1 tablespoon soy sauce, tamari, or coconut aminos

12 cups water

Store-bought chicken broth is good, but homemade is better. In addition to having more flavor and the option of customizing the broth to your liking, making chicken broth from scratch yields delicious poached chicken to use in other recipes. Homemade broth is also a good way to ensure that it is nightshade-free. Nightshade vegetables worsen symptoms of fibromyalgia and are best avoided. For optimal flavor, do not peel your aromatic vegetables. Instead, just give them a quick scrub before tossing them in the pot. This recipe does cook for longer than 30 minutes, which is necessary to extract the chicken flavor, but the cooking time is passive.

1. In a large pot, combine the chicken, onion, garlic, celery, parsley, salt, and pepper.

2. Pour in the soy sauce.

3. Bring to a boil, reduce to a simmer, cover, and let simmer for 1 hour and 30 minutes.

4. Once cool enough to handle, remove the chicken from the pot and shred.

5. Strain the liquid and use immediately, or let cool and freeze to use at a later time.

Tip: Chicken broth can be refrigerated for 3 days or frozen for up to 6 months. Shredded chicken can be refrigerated for 4 days or frozen for up to 3 months.

....

Per serving (1 cup): Calories: 30; Total fat: 1g; Total carbs: 1g; Fiber: <1g; Sugar: <1g; Protein: 3g; Sodium: 160mg

SHAWARMA SEASONING

MAKE-AHEAD, ONE-POT, VEGAN

Makes ¼ cup
Prep time: 2 minutes

2 tablespoons ground cumin

2 teaspoons ground turmeric

1 teaspoon ground cinnamon

1 teaspoon ground ginger

1 teaspoon ground coriander

1 teaspoon freshly ground
   black pepper

¼ teaspoon ground cardamom

Shawarma seasoning is a spice cabinet must-have. Its complexity is sublime, yet it pairs well with anything from shawarma to an omelet and even sautéed vegetables. It is smoky, complex, and a touch sweet, with a bold kick, notes of freshness, and so much more. Store-bought blends often contain nightshades, which may aggravate pain or inflammation. This seasoning is nightshade-free, consists of anti-inflammatory spices, and is high in antioxidants.

Add the spices to a small jar. Shake well and seal with a tight-fitting lid. Use in your favorite recipes.

Tip: Swap the cardamom for ground cloves if you prefer a spice blend with a peppery pine-like flavor. The spice blend can be stored at room temperature for several months.

Per serving (1 tablespoon): Calories: 21; Total fat: 1g; Total carbs: 4g; Fiber: 1g; Sugar: <1g; Protein: 1g; Sodium: 6mg

PICKLED AVOCADOS

FIVE INGREDIENTS OR LESS, MAKE-AHEAD, ONE-POT, VEGAN

Serves 4
Prep time: 35 minutes

½ cup white vinegar

½ cup water

1 tablespoon salt

1 avocado, ripe but still firm, halved and cut into ¼-inch-thick slices

Pickles are a great way to add tangy flavorful condiments to any dish. Getting creative with brine can be fun! The combination of a creamy, just-ripe avocado with brine is unexpected and exceptional, and just the right topping for any main dish. For maximum flavor, make these the night before you want to use them.

1. In a jar, combine the vinegar, water, and salt and whisk or shake until the salt is dissolved, about 30 seconds.

2. Add the avocado slices to the jar and refrigerate for 30 minutes.

3. To serve, use a fork or tongs to gently remove the slices from the jar.

Tip: Check avocados daily for firmness. You want it to barely yield to the pressure of your hand for ideal texture. To help avocados ripen, you can put them in a brown paper bag with an apple. Ethylene gas helps avocados ripen, and apples give off this gas as they themselves ripen. Pickled avocados will keep in the refrigerator for 3 days.

Per serving: Calories: 57; Total fat: 5g; Total carbs: 3g; Fiber: 2g; Sugar: <1g; Protein: 1g; Sodium: 887mg

ALMOND FLOUR CRACKERS

FIVE INGREDIENTS OR LESS, FREEZER-FRIENDLY, MAKE-AHEAD, VEGAN

Serves 5
Prep time: 7 minutes
Cook time: 15 minutes

½ cup almond flour

½ cup ground flaxseed meal

⅓ cup vegan Parmesan cheese (optional)

1 teaspoon garlic powder

½ teaspoon salt

½ cup water

A 2013 study published in the European Journal of Nutrition *found that when subjects increased their consumption of almonds they decreased the oxidative stress and inflammatory markers in their blood. These almond flour crackers are so easy to put together and they taste so much better than any store-bought cracker. Rolling out the dough does not take too much time, but if you are having pain in your hands you might want to save this for another day.*

1. Preheat the oven to 375°F.

2. In a bowl, mix the almond flour, flaxseed meal, vegan Parmesan (if using), garlic powder, and salt. Add the water and mix until combined. Set aside for 5 minutes, or until the water is absorbed and you can form a ball with the dough.

3. Cut a sheet of parchment paper to the size of a baking sheet. Place the dough on the parchment paper and cover with plastic wrap. Use a rolling pin on top of the plastic wrap to roll out the dough until it is ⅛-inch thick. Remove the plastic wrap.

4. Use a butter knife to score the dough into squares, without cutting completely through to the paper. Place the parchment paper with the rolled-out dough on a baking sheet and bake for 15 minutes.

5. After the crackers are completely cooled, break them apart into squares and store in an airtight container in the refrigerator for up to 1 week.

Tip: You can substitute nutritional yeast for the Parmesan cheese if you like, or omit it altogether. You can also sprinkle spices on top of the crackers before baking for extra flavors. These crackers are great with guacamole or hummus, or topped with the vegan cheese from the Almond "Feta Cheese" Wheel (page 112).

Per serving: Calories: 130; Total fat: 10g; Total carbs: 6g; Fiber: 5g; Sugar: <1g; Protein: 6g; Sodium: 240mg

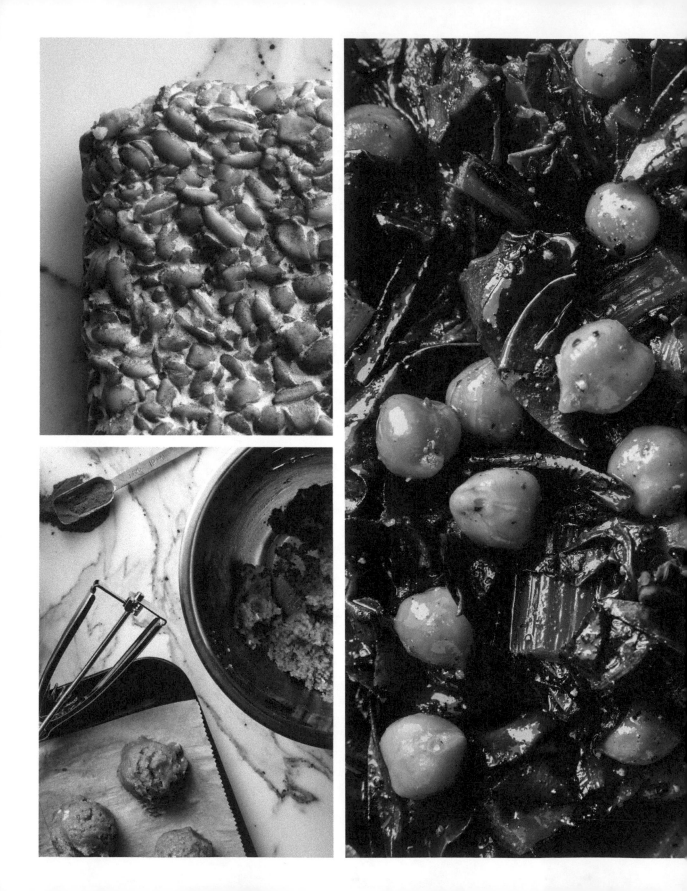

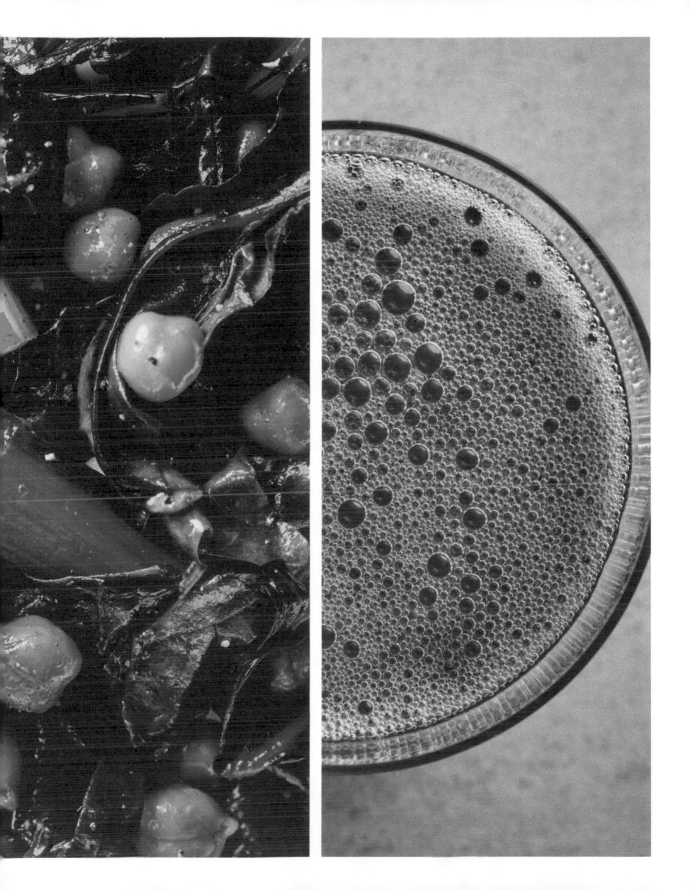

MEASUREMENT CONVERSIONS

Volume Equivalents	US STANDARD	US STANDARD (OUNCES)	METRIC (APPROXIMATE)
Liquid	2 tablespoons	1 fl. oz.	30 mL
	¼ cup	2 fl. oz.	60 mL
	½ cup	4 fl. oz.	120 mL
	1 cup	8 fl. oz.	240 mL
	1½ cups	12 fl. oz.	355 mL
	2 cups or 1 pint	16 fl. oz.	475 mL
	4 cups or 1 quart	32 fl. oz.	1 L
	1 gallon	128 fl. oz.	4 L
Dry	⅛ teaspoon	—	0.5 mL
	¼ teaspoon	—	1 mL
	½ teaspoon	—	2 mL
	¾ teaspoon	—	4 mL
	1 teaspoon	—	5 mL
	1 tablespoon	—	15 mL
	¼ cup	—	59 mL
	⅓ cup	—	79 mL
	½ cup	—	118 mL
	⅔ cup	—	156 mL
	¾ cup	—	177 mL
	1 cup	—	235 mL
	2 cups or 1 pint	—	475 mL
	3 cups	—	700 mL
	4 cups or 1 quart	—	1 L
	½ gallon	—	2 L
	1 gallon	—	4 L

Oven Temperatures

FAHRENHEIT	CELSIUS (APPROXIMATE)
250°F	120°C
300°F	150°C
325°F	165°C
350°F	180°C
375°F	190°C
400°F	200°C
425°F	220°C
450°F	230°C

Weight Equivalents

US STANDARD	METRIC (APPROXIMATE)
½ ounce	15 g
1 ounce	30 g
2 ounces	60 g
4 ounces	115 g
8 ounces	225 g
12 ounces	340 g
16 ounces or 1 pound	455 g

RESOURCES

Beyond Meat (BeyondMeat.com). If you prefer being a vegan but want some vegetarian "meat," try Beyond Meat products. Their products are pea protein–based and soy-free for anyone avoiding soy products.

Cronometer (Cronometer.com). If you would like to track your food intake and look for patterns to find an elusive food trigger, try this app. You can input foods and use the notes section to write in any symptoms you are experiencing. After a few weeks, analyze your data or hand over the info to a registered dietitian skilled in food-trigger analysis.

Fibro Food Fairy (FibroFoodFairy.co.uk). Charlie Davies, a fellow fibromyalgia warrior, has built up a fantastic website complete with helpful information and great recipes.

Just Egg (ju.st/en-us). Try this product for a fried or scrambled egg substitute.

Lakanto products (Lakanto.com/collections/shop-products). Eliminating sugar and artificial sweeteners can be difficult. Some of the best all-natural alternatives are the products by Lakanto. They have a granulated "sugar" made from monk fruit, and also offer a maple syrup alternative.

Liptan, Ginevra. *The Fibro Manual* (2016). A great book to use as a reference guide by a physician and fibromyalgia warrior. This book is comprehensive and evidence based.

Pain Resource (PainResource.com). Visit this site for excellent evidence-based information regarding all things pain.

REFERENCES

Baenas, Nieves, et al. "Broccoli Sprouts in Analgesia–Preclinical *In Vivo* Studies." *Food & Function* 8, no. 1 (January 25, 2017): 167–176. doi: 10.1039/c6fo01489e.

Choy, E., S. Perrot, T. Leon, et al. "A Patient Survey of the Impact of Fibromyalgia and the Journey to Diagnosis," *BMC Health Services Research* 10, no. 102 (2010), doi.org/10.1186/1472-6963-10-102.

Daily, James W., et al. "Efficacy of Turmeric Extracts and Curcumin for Alleviating the Symptoms of Joint Arthritis: A Systematic Review and Meta-Analysis of Randomized Clinical Trials." *Journal of Medicinal Food* 19, no. 8 (August 1, 2016): 717–29. doi:10.1089/jmf.2016.3705.

Di Pierro, F., et al. "A Naturally-Inspired, Curcumin-Based Lecithin Formulation (Meriva® Formulated as the Finished Product Algocur®) Alleviates the Osteo-Muscular Pain Conditions in Rugby Players." *European Review for Medical and Pharmacological Sciences* 21, no. 21 (November 2017): 4935–40, EuropeanReview.org/article/13738.

Hermsdorff, Helen Hermana M., et al. "A Legume-Based Hypocaloric Diet Reduces Proinflammatory Status and Improves Metabolic Features in Overweight/Obese Subjects." *European Journal of Nutrition* 50, no. 1 (February 2011): 61–9. doi: 10.1007/s00394-010-0115-x.

Holton, Kathleen. "The Role of Diet in the Treatment of Fibromyalgia." *Pain Management* 6, no. 4 (May 2016): 317–20. doi: 10.2217/pmt-2016-0019.

Kaartinen, K., et al. "Vegan Diet Alleviates Fibromyalgia Symptoms." *Scandinavian Journal of Rheumatology* 29, no. 5 (2000): 308–13. doi: 10.1080/030097400447697.

Kadioglu, Onat, et al. "Kaempferol Is an Anti-Inflammatory Compound with Activity towards NF-KB Pathway Proteins." *Anticancer Research* 35, no. 5 (May 2015): 2645–50. PubMed.ncbi.nlm.nih.gov/25964540.

Kelley, Darshan S., et al. "A Review of the Health Benefits of Cherries." *Nutrients* 10, no. 3 (March 17, 2018): 368. doi:10.3390/nu10030368.

Kuptniratsaikul, V., et al. "Efficacy and Safety of *Curcuma domestica* Extracts Compared with Ibuprofen in Patients with Knee Osteoarthritis: A Multicenter Study." *Clinical Interventions in Aging* 9 (March 20, 2014): 451–8. doi: 10.2147/CIA.S58535.

Liu, Jen-Fang, et al. "The Effect of Almonds on Inflammation and Oxidative Stress in Chinese Patients with Type 2 Diabetes Mellitus: A Randomized Crossover Controlled Feeding Trial." *European Journal of Nutrition* 52, no. 3 (April 2013): 927–35. doi: 10.1007/s00394-012-0400-y.

Martínez-Rodríguez, Alejandro, et al. "Effects of Lacto-Vegetarian Diet and Stabilization Core Exercises on Body Composition and Pain in Women with Fibromyalgia: Randomized Controlled Trial." *Nutricion Hospitalaria* 35, no. 2 (March 2018): 392–9. doi: 10.20960/nh.1341.

Marum, Ana Paula, Catia Moreira, Fernando Saraiva, Pablo Tomas-Carus, and Catarina Sousa-Guerreiro. "A Low Fermentable Oligo-di-mono Saccharides and Polyols (FODMAP) Diet Reduced Pain and Improve Daily Life in Fibromyalgia Patients." *Scandinavian Journal of Pain* 13, no. 1 (October 1, 2016): 166–72. doi.org/10.1016/j.sjpain.2016.07.004.

Selvaraju, Subash, et al. "Neuroprotective Effects of Berry Fruits on Neurodegenerative Diseases." *Neural Regeneration Research* 9, no. 16 (August 15, 2014): 1557–66. doi: 10.4103/1673-5374.139483.

Townsend, Brigitte E., et al. "Dietary Broccoli Mildly Improves Neuroinflammation in Aged Mice but Does Not Reduce Lipopolysaccharide-Induced Sickness Behavior." *Nutrition Research* 34, no. 11 (November 2014): 990–9. doi: 10.1016/j.nutres.2014.10.001.

Yilmaz, Naside, and Emine Kiyak. "The Effects of Local Cold Application on Fibromyalgia Pain." *International Journal of Rheumatic Diseases* 20, no. 8 (April 17, 2017): 929–34. doi.org/10.1111/1756-185X.13078.

Yuichiro, Honda, et al. "Effects of Physical-Agent Pain Relief Modalities for Fibromyalgia Patients: A Systematic Review and Meta-Analysis of Randomized Controlled Trials." *Pain Research and Management* 2018 (October 1, 2018): 2930632. doi.org/10.1155/2018/2930632.

INDEX

ACKNOWLEDGMENTS

This book was written during the outbreak of COVID-19, when the world shut down, and my world was limited to everything that was inside my home. To my incredible husband, Alan: Your calm demeanor kept me grounded and helped me continue forward in the midst of chaos. Even when you contracted the dreaded virus, you continued to be my source of comfort, taking care of me when I, too, fell ill.

A huge debt of gratitude is owed to my amazing children, Juliet, Elizabeth, Steven, and Sophia, for being so understanding during this quarantine book-writing process. From pitching in with laundry to cooking meals and monitoring one another in online school, you really made this book a group effort. And just FYI, any perceived yelling that went on during the shelter-in-place orders was a figment of your very active imaginations.

Many thanks to my mother, Helen, and my sisters, Sandy and Sara, for their text support and meme exchanges during my most difficult moments. Your words of encouragement helped me tremendously.

Of course, I would like to thank everyone at Callisto. Joe Cho, thank you for believing in me, and Nadina Persaud, thank you for your edits, comments, and cheerleading.

ABOUT THE AUTHOR

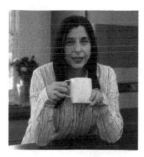 **Bonnie Nasar, RDN,** has been a dietitian for over 20 years. She currently maintains a private practice via telenutrition, specializing in chronic pain and its associated conditions. She lives in New Jersey, where she spends a lot of time drinking tea and cooking meals for her husband and four children.

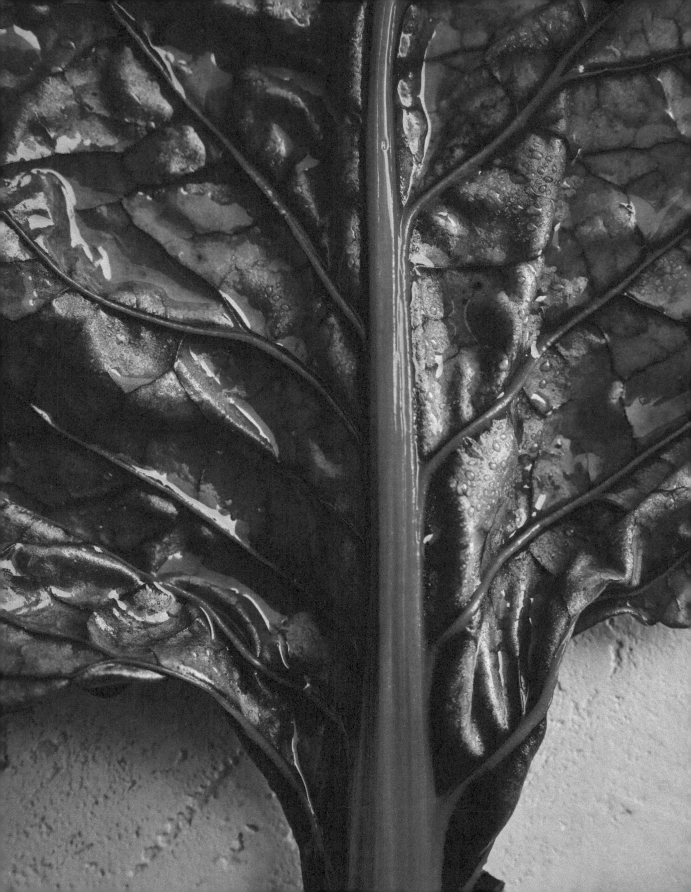

Printed in the USA
CPSIA information can be obtained
at www.ICGtesting.com
LVHW081657301123
764704LV00004B/66

9 781647 396862